Essential Measurements in Pediatric Musculoskeletal Imaging

Paolo Simoni
Maria Pilar Aparisi Gómez
Editors

Essential Measurements in Pediatric Musculoskeletal Imaging

Springer

Editors
Paolo Simoni
Pediatric Imaging Department
Reine Fabiola Children's
University Hospital, Université
Libre de Bruxelles
Brussels, Belgium

Maria Pilar Aparisi Gómez
Department of Radiology
Auckland City Hospital
Te Toka Tumai Auckland
Auckland, New Zealand

Department of Radiology
IMSKE
Valencia, Spain

ISBN 978-3-031-17734-7 ISBN 978-3-031-17735-4 (eBook)
https://doi.org/10.1007/978-3-031-17735-4

This Springer imprint is published by the registered company Springer Nature Switzerland AG
The registered company address is: Gewerbestrasse 11, 6330 Cham, Switzerland

To all children, especially those with limited or no access to healthcare, with the wish for a better future.

Paolo Simoni

To my parents, my love, my family. You are my points of reference.
To Pancho and Evie, who will never be able to read this book, or understand distances.
What I owe you is unmeasurable.

Maria Pilar Aparisi Gómez

Foreword

We are delighted and feel privileged to be able to write a foreword for this new and timely book on *Essential Measurements in Pediatric Musculoskeletal Imaging*, edited by our good friends, Paolo Simoni and Maria Pilar Aparisi Gómez, with a series of contributors that includes many distinguished experts of the pediatric musculoskeletal radiology community, most of them members of the European Musculoskeletal Radiology Society (ESSR). Measurements represent one of the key parameters in radiology and an essential part for distinguishing normal from pathologic conditions. This is particularly true in the musculoskeletal system of children and adolescents where the growing skeleton and the timing and status of bone maturation may introduce additional variables influencing the correct interpretation of imaging findings.

Essential Measurements in Pediatric Musculoskeletal Imaging is an invaluable text comprising 12 chapters that encompass the whole children age period from in utero to late adolescence following a regional-based approach. Each of the chapters is extensively illustrated with figures that form the background and reference for each measurement. When needed, diagnostic images have been complemented with very clear schematic drawings for better understanding of complex procedures.

Overall, the book is schematic, extremely readable for consultation, and its illustrations help in the clarification of points made in the text. It will be of great practical value not only for pediatric radiologists or musculoskeletal radiologists whose practice includes pediatric imaging but also for pediatricians and pediatric orthopedic surgeons providing all of these specialists with state-of-the-art information on a field that has been largely ignored despite its relevant clinical impact.

We would like to thank the editors and the authors and congratulate them most sincerely for their superb efforts that have resulted in this outstanding work. In the end, *Essential Measurements in Pediatric Musculoskeletal Imaging* may be a volume of extreme practical usefulness in the field of pediatric musculoskeletal radiology and we are confident it will remain a classic for years to come.

Carlo Martinoli
(ESSR president 2022 - 2023)
Department of Health Sciences (DISSAL),
University of Genoa, Genova, Italy.
IRCCS Ospedale Policlinico San Martino,
Genova, Italy.

Eva Llopis
(ESSR president 2021 - 2022)
Hospital de la Ribera, Valencia, Spain
Department of Radiology, IMSKE, Valencia, Spain

Preface

The practice of pediatric musculoskeletal radiology relies on the adequate knowledge of anatomy, physiology, pathology, and background genetics of the child and adolescent, but also, like any other discipline of pediatric imaging, on a good dose of training and experience. Complex, challenging, and atypical cases abound in pediatric imaging, while robust guidelines, appropriateness criteria, and studies on large populations are notoriously limited or absent.

The greatest challenge for radiologists and health professionals involved in pediatric musculoskeletal imaging is to combine expertise with modern evidence-based approaches.

In the context of evidence-based medicine, the focus of imaging is shifting from simple description towards quantification, with measurements becoming more important to make the diagnosis and distinguish the normal from the pathological.

In pediatrics, most measurements change over time and are dependent on development and gender. Besides, the peak of puberty is different in boys and girls, so single reference values are not sufficient, and instead normative values for patient groups are necessary for an accurate diagnosis.

It is important to highlight that common measurements used in adults may not be validated for the pediatric population. Performing searches and contrasting evidence on measurements that have been validated for children may be an arduous task in the context of increasing reporting volumes, interrupting normal workflow.

For this reason, this text summarizes, in a comprehensive but easy to refer way, the measurements that are most commonly used in clinical practice and have been validated in pediatric populations. Examples are presented on real diagnostic images to allow the most practical demonstration.

Beyond measurements, some normal developmental appearances and variants of anatomical structures are discussed, when the correct interpretation of the images depends on the presence of these.

In some cases, measurements that have not been validated in children but are used in clinical practice in pediatrics are included in the text, with an appropriate note to interpret the measurements with caution.

There is the expectation that this book will serve as a valid tool to speed up diagnosis and optimize assessment, potentially reducing unnecessary diagnostic steps that may involve radiation in children.

It is humbly hoped by the editors and authors that this book will find a place among the desktop texts that colleagues can refer to frequently and with confidence.

Brussels, Belgium — Paolo Simoni
Auckland, New Zealand — Maria Pilar Aparisi Gómez

Acknowledgments

This work has been compiled by some members of the Pediatric Subcommittee of the European Society of Skeletal Radiology, which is formed by an international team of radiologists with predominant experience and expertise in pediatric musculoskeletal imaging.

The authors were entrusted with the difficult task of succinctly compiling the available measurements that prove important in practice, often based on limited evidence on literature, which required a particularly careful and critical analysis.

They deserve our heartfelt gratitude and sincere acknowledgement for the hard work done.

Contents

In-Utero

Maria Pilar Aparisi Gómez, Sheryl Watkin, and Alberto Bazzocchi

Introduction: Prenatal Ultrasound

Development

The evaluation of fetuses in the second trimester for the detection of abnormalities represents a standard of care in many communities [1].

M. P. Aparisi Gómez (✉)
Department of Radiology, Auckland City Hospital, Te Toka Tumai Auckland, Auckland, New Zealand

Department of Radiology, IMSKE, Valencia, Spain
e-mail: pilara@adhb.govt.nz

S. Watkin
Department of Radiology, National Women's Ultrasound, Auckland City Hospital, Te Toka Tumai Auckland, Auckland, New Zealand

A. Bazzocchi
Diagnostic and Interventional Radiology, IRCCS Istituto Ortopedico Rizzoli, Bologna, Italy

P. Simoni, M. P. Aparisi Gómez (eds.), *Essential Measurements in Pediatric Musculoskeletal Imaging*,
https://doi.org/10.1007/978-3-031-17735-4_1

Morphogenesis of the skeletal systems occurs from the third to the eighth week intra utero, and therefore, prenatal diagnosis of some skeletal disorders is possible.

Week	Development	Activity
8	Limb buds, clavicle, mandible	
9	Femur, humerus	Body movements
10	Tibia/fibula, radius/ulna	
11–12	Accurate measurements can be performed	Limb movement
20	Epiphyseal ossification centers visible (long bones)	

Summarized from Chitty and Altman [2] and van Zalen-Sprock et al. [3]

The appendicular and axial skeleton follow a pattern of endochondral ossification. The calvarium, portions of the clavicle, and pubis follow a pattern of membranous ossification [4].

The measurement of fetal limbs has been used to date pregnancies and constitutes and important part of the assessment of fetal anatomy [5].

The femur length is the most commonly used limb measurement and is also included in the regular growth scans, as one of the parameters to assess growth, and to obtain an estimate on fetal weight [6]. The increase in size of long bones is linear throughout gestation [7].

Imaging Workup When a Skeletal Dysplasia Is Suspected in Utero (Prenatal Ultrasound)

When the femoral or humeral measurements are less than the fifth percentile or less than two standard deviations (SD) from the mean in the second trimester, fetal medicine referral and complete evaluation of the skeleton should be made.

When measurements of the long bones are less than three SD from the mean, suspicion of skeletal dysplasia should be very high, especially if the head circumference is above the 75th centile.

Specific views to obtain in the suspicion of skeletal dysplasia	
All long bones	Length measurement
	Shape
	Echogenicity
	Femur-to-foot ratio
Other bones	Scapula
	Clavicle
	Mandible
Abdominal	Circumference measurement
Chest	Circumference measurement
Fetal cranium	Biparietal diameter measurement
	Occipitofrontal diameter measurement
	Head circumference measurement
Facial profile	Glabellar bossing
	Flattened nasal ridge
	Assessment of micrognathia
Vertebral bodies	Number Shape
Hands and feet	Extra digits Missing digits Malformations
Mineralization	Calvarium Skeleton Ectopic mineralization

The accuracy of diagnosis of dysplasias in prenatal ultrasound ranges between 40% and 60% [8, 9]; therefore, subsequent radiological evaluation (or in cases of demise autopsy and histomorphic analysis) is very important.

The obtention of an accurate diagnosis is important, to offer counseling to avoid the possibility of recurrence (many dysplasias have a high recurrence risk) [10].

Low-dose and ultralow-dose CT allow the exquisite depiction of fetal bones and the possibility of complete 3D rendering of the skeleton. Images can be rotated in space and postprocessed to focus on sections and obtain adequate detail. This is an important advantage with respect to dedicated ultrasound, in which the maternal habitus and the position of the fetus have a great impact on visualization.

Assessment of Characteristics of Long Bones

Bone Length

- The bones are measured in a plane as close as the orthogonal plane to the ultrasound beam.
- The full length of the bone has to be visualized, and the view should not be obscured by shadowing from adjacent body parts [7].
- Calipers are placed from the greater trochanter to the end of the ossified shaft (femur) (Fig. 1a, b). End-to-end of ossified shafts in other bones (Fig. 2a–d).

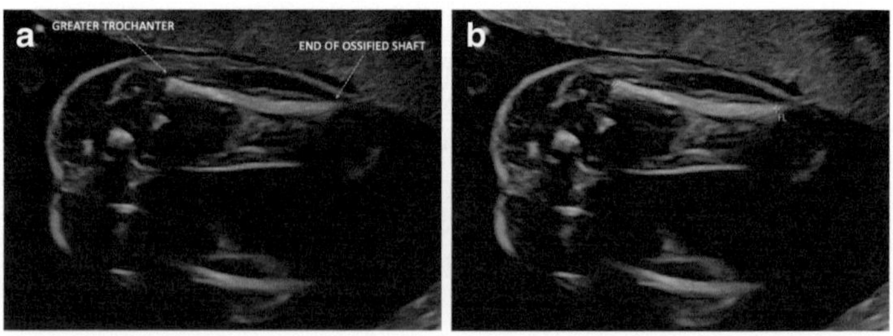

Figure 1 (**a**, **b**) Femur length measurement (landmarks)

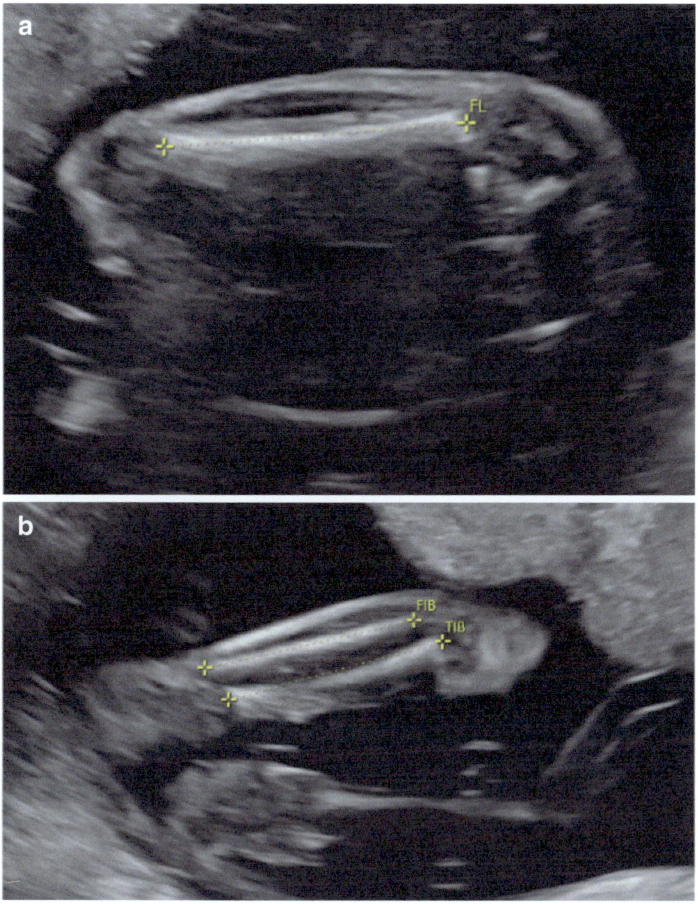

FIGURE 2 Measurements of long bones. (**a**) Femur measurement. (**b**) Tibia and fibula measurement. (**c**) Humerus measurement. (**d**) Radius and ulna measurement

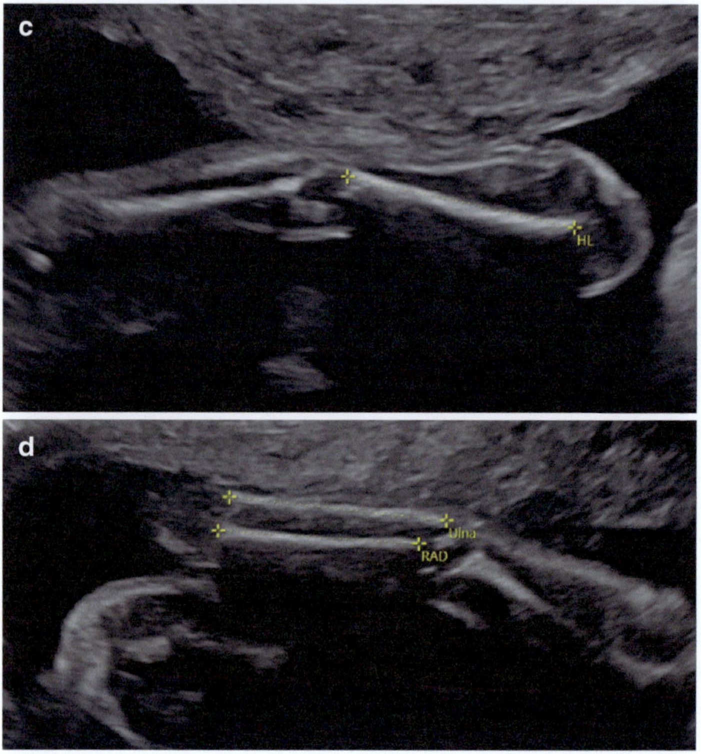

FIGURE 2 (continued)

Type of shortening	Involvement	
Micromelia	Entire limb	
Rhizomelia[a]	Proximal segment	Femur, humerus
Mesomelia[a]	Intermediate segment	Tibia, fibula, radius, ulna
Acromelia	Distal segment	Hands, feet

[a]The diagnosis of rhizomelia or mesomelia requires comparison of the length of the bones of the leg or forearm (tibia/fibula and radius/ulna) with those of the thigh and arm (femur and humerus). Plotting against normal values (population charts) is helpful to determine whether both segments may be involved [1]

- The femur-to-foot ratio approaches 1.0 throughout gestation (in our experience, the foot is almost always slightly larger than the femur) (Fig. 3). Many skeletal dysplasias show obvious disproportion of the femur-to-foot ratio: the dysplasias in which rhizomelia is predominant will show <1.0 femur-to-foot ratio [11].
- The foot is measured in the plantar view, from the heel to the end of the longest toe [2] (Fig. 4a, b).
- The more severe the reduction, the earlier it can be detected:
  - 16–18 weeks—severe limb reductions (osteogenesis imperfecta type II, achondrogenesis, thanatophoric dysplasia, diastrophic dysplasia, chondroectodermal dysplasia);
  - 22–24 weeks—less severe reductions (achondroplasia) [1].

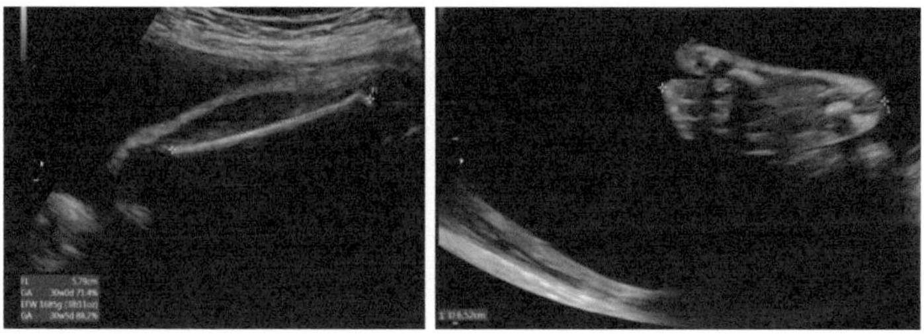

FIGURE 3 Femur-to-foot ratio

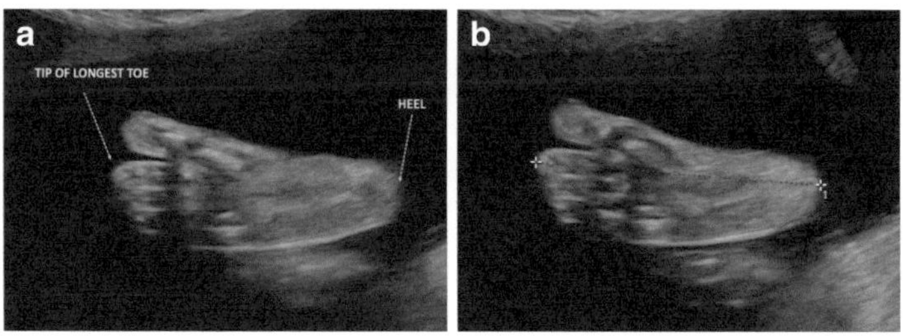

FIGURE 4 (**a**, **b**) Foot measurement (landmarks)

Isolated reduction of limbs is often inherited as part of a syndrome: Holt-Oram, Fanconi pancytopenia, and thrombocytopenia with absent radii.

- Amelia—complete absence of an extremity.
- Acheiria—absence of the hand.
- Phocomelia—absence of proximal segments: seal limb.
- Aplasia—hypoplasia of the radius or ulna.

Other causes are amniotic bands, exposure to thalidomide, and caudal regression.

Bone Shape

A small degree of curvature of the femur is a normal finding.

- Bowing: campomelic dysplasia, thanatophoric dwarfism, osteogenesis imperfecta (autosomal dominant), achondrogenesis, and hypophosphatasia.
- Fractures and callus formation: osteogenesis imperfecta (autosomal dominant), achondrogenesis, and hypophosphatasia [12].

Echogenicity

When the bones are hypomineralized, the echogenicity on ultrasound is be reduced.

Hypomineralization can be seen in conditions such as osteogenesis imperfecta, hypophosphatasia, and achondrogenesis [12].

Evaluation of Hands and Feet

- Polydactyly—more than five digits.
  - Postaxial if the additional digits are on the ulnar/fibular aspect.
  - Preaxial if they are on the radial/tibial aspect.

- Brachydactyly—missing fingers.
- Syndactyly—fusion of soft tissues or bones of adjacent digits.
- Clinodactyly—deviation of the fingers.
- Disproportion—between the hands and feet and other parts of the limb.
- Deformities—equinovarus (talipes) [13].

Evaluation of Fetal Movements

Limitation of flexion or extension of the limbs may be associated to arthrogryposis and multiple pterygium syndrome [14].

Evaluation of the Fetal Head

Many dysplasias, some of them severe, involve abnormalities of the shape or ossification of the skull bones.

Most dysplasias with a prenatal onset demonstrate a relative disproportion of the skeletal measurements compared to the measurements of the fetal head [15].

- Head measurements are obtained in a symmetric axial plane, at the level of the thalami and the cavum septum pellucidum (the cerebellum should not be included in the plane) (Fig. 5a).
  - Biparietal diameter: calipers are placed at the outer edge of the near calvarial wall and the inner edge of the far calvarial wall (Fig. 5b).
  - Head circumference: ellipse should be drawn around the outside of the calvarium (Fig. 5c).
- The face also needs to be evaluated: hypertelorism, micrognathia, short philtrum, and abnormal morphology or location of the ears.

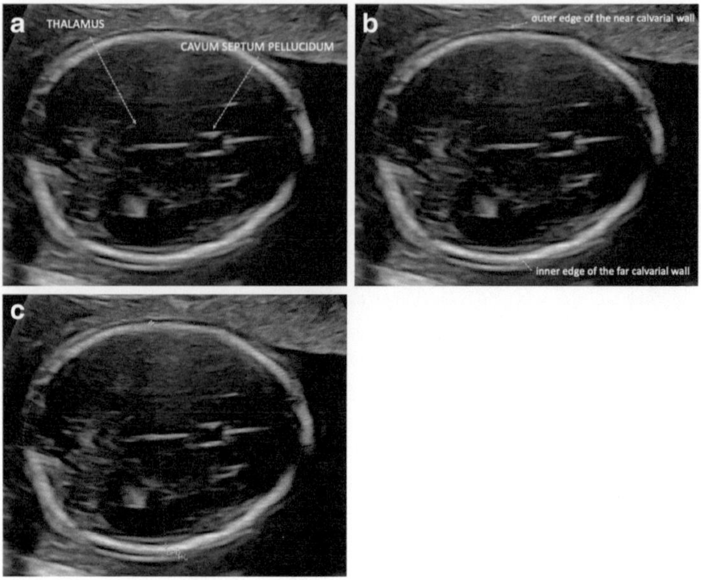

FIGURE 5 (**a**, **b**, **c**) Head measurements (landmarks and measurements)

Abdominal Circumference

Abdominal circumference is measured at a level including the fetal stomach, umbilical vein, and adrenal glands (Fig. 6a). The descending aorta should appear in true cross section (completely round). Kidneys should not be visible. The calipers should be placed in the skin line (Fig. 6b).

Evaluation of the Fetal Thorax

Severe skeletal dysplasias are associated with a small thorax, which is linked to pulmonary hypoplasia, and associated with neonatal death [16].

- The bony thoracic circumference is measured at the level of the four-chamber view. The whole thorax should be vis-

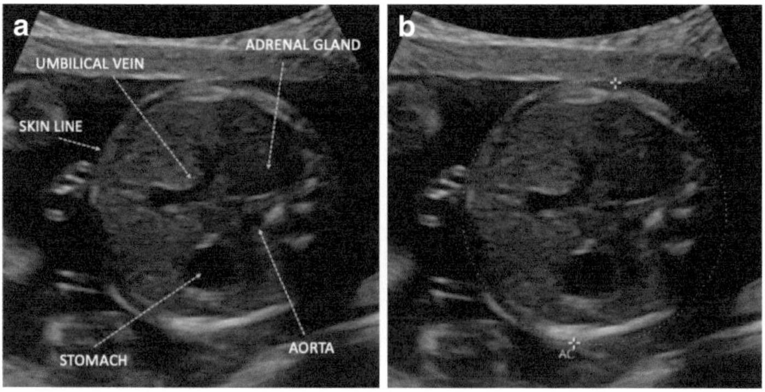

FIGURE 6 (**a, b**) Abdominal circumference measurement (landmarks and measurements)

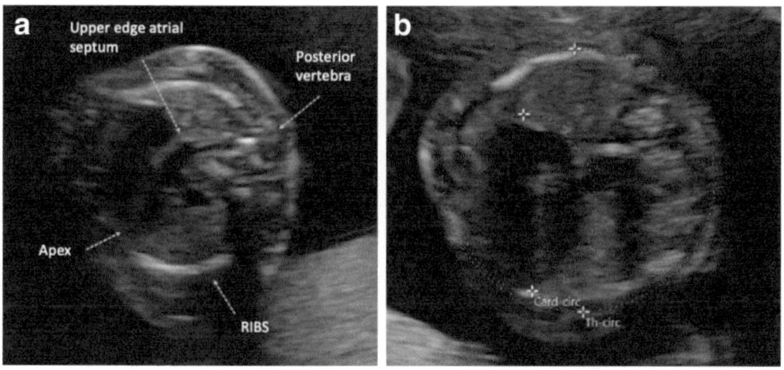

FIGURE 7 (**a, b**) Thoracic measurements (landmarks and measurements of the cardiac and thoracic circumferences)

ible in the screen, with ribs on both sides, and no abdominal contents. The points of reference for the circumference are the anterior thoracic wall and the posterior edge of the fetal vertebra. Measurements are performed with the heart in diastole. Reference points for the heart are the cardiac apex and the upper edge of the atrial septum [17, 18] (Fig. 7).

Determination of Lethality

One of the most important tasks for prenatal ultrasound in the context of a skeletal abnormality is to determine the neonatal or infantile lethality of the condition.

Lethality is normally linked to small chest circumference and subsequent pulmonary hypoplasia, which leads to early postnatal death. Not all skeletal dysplasias with small chests will result in immediate death.

Strongly linked to lethality:

- Chest-to-abdominal circumference ratio <0.6 [19] (Fig. 8).
- Femur length-to-abdominal circumference ratio <0.16 [20].
- Evaluate the occurrence of other abnormalities in other systems (heart, urogenital).
- Other markers of lethality:
  - Severe long bone shortening (more than three SD from mean).
  - Hydrops.
  - Markedly decreased bone echogenicity and prominent bowing or fractures [16, 21].

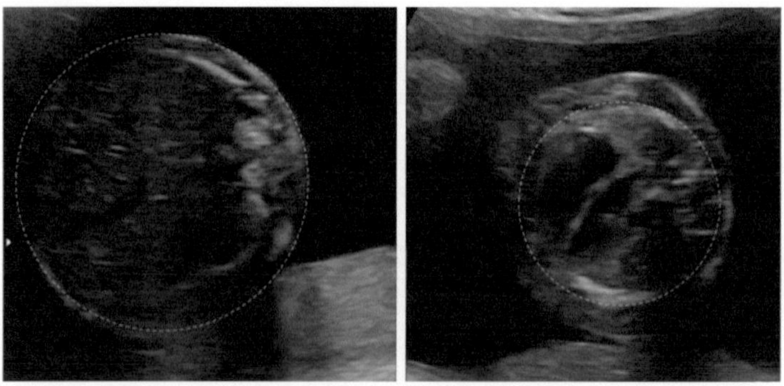

FIGURE 8 Comparison in size of abdomen and thorax

Imaging Workup When a Skeletal Dysplasia Is Suspected Postnatally (Radiographs)

If a skeletal dysplasia is suspected, a skeletal survey needs to be performed. This consists of a series of radiographs that will sample the structure and morphology of a wide range of bone structures.

Early radiographs are very useful. The ideal age for recognition of most dysplasias is before the closing of the growth epiphyses. After this, radiological diagnosis may be impossible [22].

Ideally, the skeletal survey should include [23, 24]:

- Skull (AP and lateral).
- Thoracolumbar spine (AP and lateral).
- Chest (AP).
- Pelvis (AP).
- One upper limb (AP).
- One lower limb (AP).
- Left hand (AP)*.

*The left hand is included to assess bone age. This is important in some cases in which it is necessary to relativize findings to the stage of normal growth [25]. Bone age may also be obtained from the foot and ankle, or the knee (especially in children younger then 2 years).

Specific Considerations

- If the limbs are visibly asymmetrical, or if there is the suspicion of epiphyseal involvement or stippling, views of both limbs (upper and lower) should be obtained for more accurate assessment.
- May be useful to obtain dedicated views (dedicated projections) that would better display the abnormality.

- Radiological surveys (and previous imaging) from affected family members may give an insight on future appearances, aid with diagnosis and prognosis, and help with the pattern of inheritance.
- Serial evaluation. This should not be done too early though—most centers would not repeat in less than 12 months [24].

References

1. Pilu G, Nicolaides KH. Diagnosis of fetal abnormalities: the 18–23-week scan. New York: Parthenon Publication Group; 1999.
2. Chitty LS, Altman DG. Charts of fetal size: limb bones. BJOG. 2002;109:919–29. https://doi.org/10.1111/j.1471-0528.2002.01022.x.
3. van Zalen-Sprock RM, Brons JT, van Vugt JM, et al. Ultrasonographic and radiologic visualization of the developing embryonic skeleton. Ultrasound Obstet Gynecol. 1997;9:392–7. https://doi.org/10.1046/j.1469-0705.1997.09060392.x.
4. Olsen BR, Reginato AM, Wang W. Bone development. Annu Rev Cell Dev Biol. 2000;16:191–220. https://doi.org/10.1146/annurev.cellbio.16.1.191.
5. Altman DG, Chitty LS. Charts of fetal size: 1 methodology. Br J Obstet Gynaecol. 1994;101:29–34. https://doi.org/10.1111/j.1471-0528.1994.tb13006.x.
6. Chitty LS, Altman DG, Henderson A, Campbell S. Charts of fetal size: 4 femur length. Br J Obstet Gynaecol. 1994;101:132–5. https://doi.org/10.1111/j.1471-0528.1994.tb13078.x.
7. Exacoustos C, Rosati P, Rizzo G, Arduini D. Ultrasound measurements of fetal limb bones. Ultrasound Obstet Gynecol. 1991;1:325–30. https://doi.org/10.1046/j.1469-0705.1991.01050325.x.
8. Doray B, Favre R, Viville B, et al. Prenatal sonographic diagnosis of skeletal dysplasias. A report of 47 cases. Ann Genet. 2000;43:163–9. https://doi.org/10.1016/s0003-3995(00)01026-1.
9. Parilla BV, Leeth EA, Kambich MP, et al. Antenatal detection of skeletal dysplasias. J Ultrasound Med. 2003;22:255–8; quiz 259–261. https://doi.org/10.7863/jum.2003.22.3.255.
10. Krakow D, Williams J, Poehl M, et al. Use of three-dimensional ultrasound imaging in the diagnosis of prenatal-onset skeletal dysplasias. Ultrasound Obstet Gynecol. 2003;21:467–72. https://doi.org/10.1002/uog.111.

11. Campbell J, Henderson A, Campbell S. The fetal femur/foot length ratio: a new parameter to assess dysplastic limb reduction. Obstet Gynecol. 1988;72:181–4.
12. Thomas IH, DiMeglio LA. Advances in the classification and treatment of osteogenesis imperfecta. Curr Osteoporos Rep. 2016;14:1–9. https://doi.org/10.1007/s11914-016-0299-y.
13. Cole P, Kaufman Y, Hatef DA, Hollier LH. Embryology of the hand and upper extremity. J Craniofac Surg. 2009;20:992–5. https://doi.org/10.1097/SCS.0b013e3181abb18e.
14. Skaria P, Dahl A, Ahmed A. Arthrogryposis multiplex congenita in utero: radiologic and pathologic findings. J Matern Fetal Neonatal Med. 2019;32:502–11. https://doi.org/10.1080/14767058.2017.1381683.
15. Krakow D, Lachman RS, Rimoin DL. Guidelines for the prenatal diagnosis of fetal skeletal dysplasias. Genet Med. 2009;11:127–33. https://doi.org/10.1097/GIM.0b013e3181971ccb.
16. Savarirayan R, Rossiter JP, Hoover-Fong JE, et al. Best practice guidelines regarding prenatal evaluation and delivery of patients with skeletal dysplasia. Am J Obstet Gynecol. 2018;219:545–62. https://doi.org/10.1016/j.ajog.2018.07.017.
17. Awadh AMA, Prefumo F, Bland JM, Carvalho JS. Assessment of the intraobserver variability in the measurement of fetal cardiothoracic ratio using ellipse and diameter methods. Ultrasound Obstet Gynecol. 2006;28:53–6. https://doi.org/10.1002/uog.2813.
18. Merz E, Miric-Tesanic D, Bahlmann F, et al. Prenatal sonographic chest and lung measurements for predicting severe pulmonary hypoplasia. Prenat Diagn. 1999;19:614–9. https://doi.org/10.1002/(sici)1097-0223(199907)19:7<614::aid-pd595>3.0.co;2-p.
19. Yoshimura S, Masuzaki H, Gotoh H, et al. Ultrasonographic prediction of lethal pulmonary hypoplasia: comparison of eight different ultrasonographic parameters. Am J Obstet Gynecol. 1996;175:477–83. https://doi.org/10.1016/s0002-9378(96)70165-5.
20. Rahemtullah A, McGillivray B, Wilson RD. Suspected skeletal dysplasias: femur length to abdominal circumference ratio can be used in ultrasonographic prediction of fetal outcome. Am J Obstet Gynecol. 1997;177:864–9. https://doi.org/10.1016/S0002-9378(97)70284-9.
21. Gaffney G, Manning N, Boyd PA, et al. Prenatal sonographic diagnosis of skeletal dysplasias—a report of the diagnostic and prognostic accuracy in 35 cases. Prenat Diagn. 1998;18:357–62.
22. Kozlowski K. The radiographic clues in the diagnosis of bone dysplasias. Pediatr Radiol. 1985;15:1–3. https://doi.org/10.1007/BF02387842.

23. Dighe M, Fligner C, Cheng E, et al. Fetal skeletal dysplasia: an approach to diagnosis with illustrative cases. Radiographics. 2008;28:1061–77. https://doi.org/10.1148/rg.284075122.
24. Offiah AC, Hall CM. Radiological diagnosis of the constitutional disorders of bone. As easy as A, B, C? Pediatr Radiol. 2003;33:153–61. https://doi.org/10.1007/s00247-002-0855-8.
25. Mazzanti L, Matteucci C, Scarano E, et al. Auxological and anthropometric evaluation in skeletal dysplasias. J Endocrinol Invest. 2010;33:19–25.

Skull

Grammatina Boitsios

Abbreviations

ADI	Atlodens interval
CI	Cranial index
CT	Computed tomography
IQ	Intellectual quotient
MRI	Magnetic resonance imaging
VRT	Volume rendering technique

Introduction

The *cranium* (or skull) comprises the cranial vault (or calvarium) and the skull base.

– The *cranial vault* includes flat bones, namely, the frontal and parietal bones, the squamous part of the temporal bones, the greater wings of the sphenoid bone and the occipital bone. Cranial vault bones grow because of

G. Boitsios (✉)
Paediatric Imaging Department, Reine Fabiola Children's University Hospital, Université libre de Bruxelles, Brussels, Belgium

P. Simoni, M. P. Aparisi Gómez (eds.), *Essential Measurements in Pediatric Musculoskeletal Imaging*,
https://doi.org/10.1007/978-3-031-17735-4_2

sutural growth, remodelling and centrifugal displacement by the underlying developing brain (intramembranous ossification) [1].

- The *skull base* is divided into three compartments (the anterior, the middle and the posterior compartments) and develops with endochondral ossification. The frontal and ethmoid bones delineate the anterior skull base; the central skull base is delineated by the sphenoid and the temporal bones; and the posterior skull base is delineated by the occipital bone.

The skull protects the underlying brain and peri-cerebral spaces. The brain communicates with the cervical spine by the foramen magnum at the craniocervical junction. The skull bones are separated by sutures, dense connective tissue formed by membranous ossification, allowing the flat bones to grow. During skull growth, sutures allow spatial separation of the bones [2]. The major dural reflections are related to the site of the suture formation.

Sutures

There are six major sutures in the neonate skull (Fig. 1):

- One metopic suture, (from the Greek μέτωπον, "after the eye," or "space between the eyes"; referring to the forehead) in the midline of the frontal bones.
- Two coronal sutures (from the Latin "corona"; meaning the "crown") connecting the frontal to the parietal bones.
- One sagittal (from the Latin "sagitta"; meaning "arrow") in the midline between the two parietal bones.
- Two lambdoid sutures (from the Greek letter λ, "lambda") posteriorly between the occipital and the parietal bones.

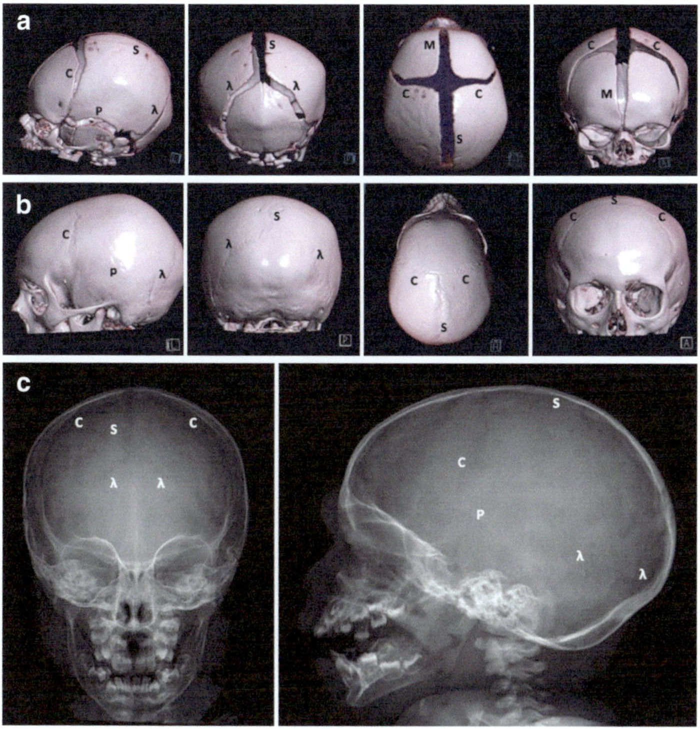

FIGURE 1 (**a**) 3D volume rendering technique (VRT) of a head CT of an 8-day-old baby boy, (**b**) VRT of a head CT of a 14-year-old boy, and (**c**) anteroposterior and lateral plain radiograph of an 18-month-old boy illustrating the cranial sutures. *C*: coronal suture, *M*: metopic suture, λ: lambdoid suture, *P*: petrosquamosal suture, *S*: sagittal suture

The metopic suture gives flexibility to the skull at the neonate's delivery, closes at the earliest 3 months and finishes at 9 months. In the general population, in 5% of cases, the metopic suture stays open (metopism) and is not to be mistaken with a vertical fracture in adults. Posteriorly, around the

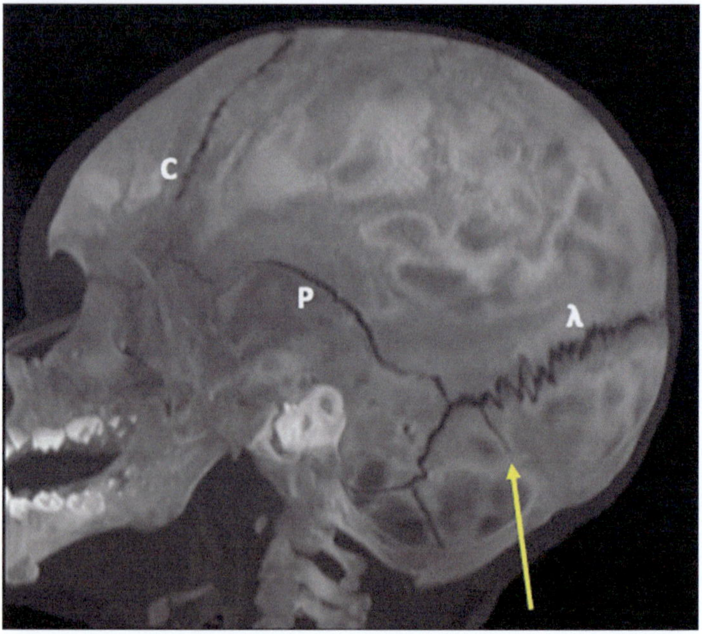

FIGURE 2 Accessory suture (yellow arrow) perpendicular to the lambdoid suture in a 6-month-old boy, normal variant. *C*: coronal suture, *λ*: lambdoid suture, *P*: petrosquamosal suture

lambdoid sutures, accessory sutures (Fig. 2) are present to provide skull elasticity for the delivery (not to be mistaken with fractures). In the lambdoid sutures, accessory bones (Wormian bones) can be found.

The sagittal suture is the most common suture involved in craniosynostosis. The average width of the sagittal suture at birth is 5.0 mm ± 0.2, narrowing significantly to 2.4 mm ± 0.1 by 1 month of age and narrowing further over time [3].

The coronal suture lies between the frontal and the parietal bones. Its average width at birth is 2.5 mm ± 0.1, narrowing significantly to 1.3 mm ± 0.1 by 1 month [3].

Apart from the major sutures, there are also minor sutures, namely, the petrosquamosal and the mendosal sutures. The two petrosquamosal sutures are located between the petrous portion and the squama of the temporal bone. The mendosal sutures (also known as the accessory occipital sutures) usually close in utero and they are present in 3% of cases [4]. Since the occipital bone rises from six ossification centres, a disturbance in the embryogenesis can lead to a persistent mendosal suture. The persistent mendosal suture is horizontal and due to incomplete fusion of the interparietal (planum occipitale, superior) and supraoccipital (planum nuchale, inferior) portions of the occipital bone. In that case, the mendosal suture runs posteriorly to the foramen magnum parallel to the skull base. The mendosal suture should not be longer than 2 cm and closed at around 6 years. If this suture is longer than 2 cm, the suspicion of a fracture in a posttraumatic event should be considered when analysing a head CT. In the parietal region, a parietal accessory suture can be incidentally found in some children. Parietal accessory sutures are vertical-oblique oriented and difficult to differentiate from fractures in young children.

Suture Closure (Table 1)

TABLE 1 Timing of closure of the cranial sutures [5]

Suture	Timing of closure
Metopic	3 months–9 months
Coronal	24 years
Sagittal	22 years
Lambdoid	26–60 years

Fontanelles

There are six fontanelles in the cranium (Fig. 3). The major fontanelles are the following:

- The anterior fontanelle (or bregma, from the Greek "βρέγμα", the "crown of the head") is located at the intersection between the coronal and the sagittal sutures, with a mean size of 2.1 cm [6] and closes at 15 to 18 months [7]. This fontanelle can bulge or depress depending on the clinical state of the child (hydrocephalus or dehydration, respectively).
- The posterior fontanelle (or lamboid) is located at the junction of the sagittal and the lambdoid sutures and closes at 2 months of age [8].

Aside from the major fontanelles, there are minor fontanelles:

- The anterolateral fontanelles, pterion (from the Greek word "πτέριον", meaning the wing), are located at the intersection of the coronal, parietosquamous and great wing of the sphenoid. The pterion close at 3 months.

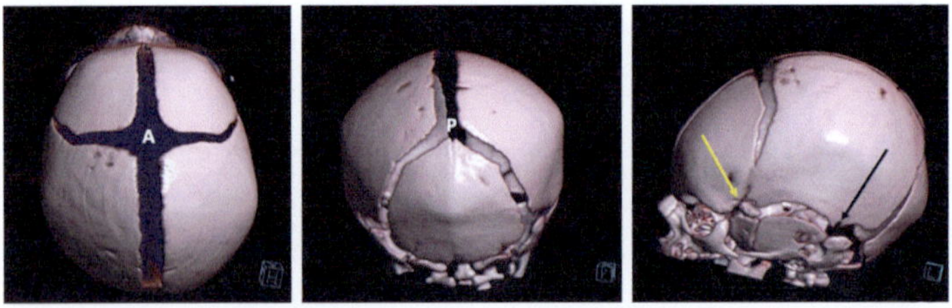

FIGURE 3 VRT reconstructions of a head CT scan of an 8-day-old newborn baby. *A*: anterior fontanelle, *P*: posterior fontanelle, yellow arrow, pterion; black arrow, asterion

- The posterolateral fontanelles, asterion (from the Greek word "ἀστέριον", meaning the star), are located at the intersection of the lambdoid, parietosquamous and mendosal sutures. The asterion closes at 24 months.

Closure Timeline of the Fontanelles (Table 2)

Apart from allowing the skull to grow with the brain, the fontanelles are also potential acoustic windows for brain sonography in neonates. The bone plates grow by producing bone at the sutures under the push of the growing brain. It is thus the brain that gives the skull its harmonious shape. Typically, until the age of 12 months, the sagittal, coronal or lambdoid sutures should appear completely open [9].

Skull Layers

From the outside to the inside, the first layer of the head is the skin and the subcutaneous fat. Then come the galea aponeurotica, the periosteum, the skull (the external table, the diploe and the internal table), the dura mater and finally, the

TABLE 2 Timing of closure of the fontanelles

Fontanelle	**Timing of closure**
Anterior (bregma)	12–18 months (median 13.8 months)
Posterior	2 months
Pterion	3 months
Asterion	24 months

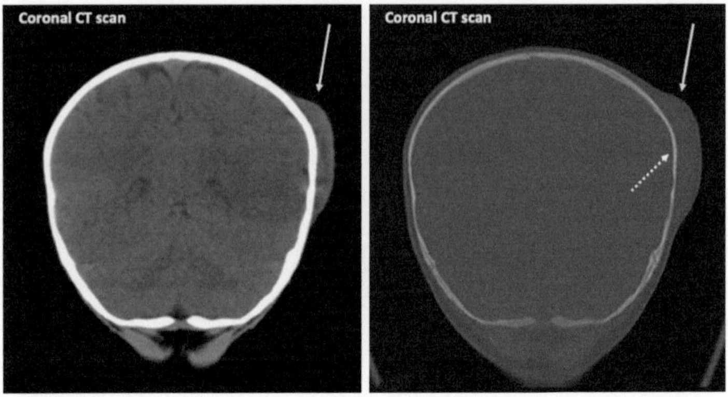

Figure 4 Coronal CT scan without contrast medium illustrating a post-traumatic subcutaneous cephalohematoma (yellow arrow) and a linear nondisplaced left parietal fracture (dotted arrow)

brain. Between each layer, the acute collections such as hematoma are named accordingly:

- *Caput succedaneum* when the hematoma is lying underneath the skin.
- Cephalohematoma is maintained by the periosteum and does not cross the sutures (Fig. 4).
- Subgaleal hematoma is located between the galea aponeurotica and the periosteum and can cross the sutures.
- Epidural hematoma is located inside the skull and exteriorly from the dura.

The skull is composed of the inner and the outer table (or diploe), separated by the diploic space. In the infants' skull base, the diploe is rich in haematopoietic marrow, richly vascularized, which can enhance on T1-weigthed sequences on brain MRI after contrast medium administration. A hypertrophic diploic space can be seen in some bone marrow disorders, such as sickle cell disease.

Many pathological conditions can cause an inhomogeneous growth of the skull: when the underlying brain is abnormal (hydrocephaly, subdural collection, Dandy-Walker malformation, Chiari I malformation), when excessive exterior pressures are applied to the skull or when there is a premature fusion of one or more cranial sutures (craniosynostosis).

Craniosynostosis

Craniosynostosis represents a premature closure of the skull sutures. The prevalence of craniosynostosis is estimated at 1 per 2500 live births. In most cases, craniosynostosis is caused by a developmental error and is then called "isolated". In 15% of cases, the premature closure of the sutures is syndromic. Of the remaining 85%, 80% are non-syndromic mono-sutural, and 20% are non-syndromic multi-sutural [10].

The cephalic index (CI) is a morphometric parameter of the skull based on the biparietal diameter (BPD) and the occipitofrontal diameter (OFD) (Fig. 5).

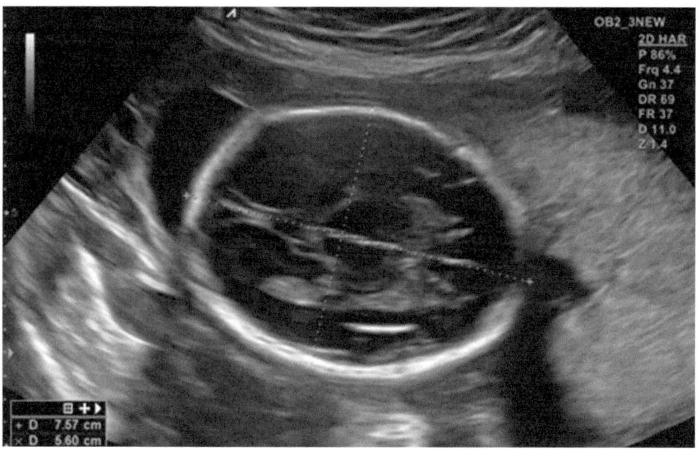

FIGURE 5 Axial plane of a prenatal brain ultrasound and the cranial index (CI = 0.74 in this example)

$$CI = \left(\frac{BPD}{OFD}\right) \times 100$$

Even though CI depends on the ethnic background, as a general rule, the normal values of the CI are between 74 and 83% (mesocephalic) [11].

The imaging workup recommended when the degree of suspicion of craniosynostosis is low or moderate is an antero-posterior and lateral radiograph of the skull. Ultrasound can be an alternative to radiographs [12]. When the skull radiographs do not exclude or confirm craniosynostosis, a CT scan of the skull must be performed. A CT scan with a 3D volume rendering (VRT) of the skull is indicated when there is a high suspicion of craniosynostosis [13]. Alternately, a "black bone" sequence on MRI can be used to detect premature closure of the sutures, without irradiation [14].

In case of craniosynostosis, surgery is indicated when there is increased intracranial pressure or an abnormal skull shape.

Non-syndromic Craniosynostosis (Table 3)

Table 3 Non-syndromic craniosynostosis, sutures involved and skull deformation

Skull deformation	**Suture involved**
Scaphocephaly (dolichocephaly)	Sagittal (CI < 75%)
Brachycephaly	Coronal or lambdoid (CI > 80%)
Trigonocephaly	Metopic
Plagiocephaly	Uni- or bicoronal
Pachycephaly	Lambdoid

Scaphocephaly (or Dolichocephaly)

Scaphocephaly (from the Greek word σκάφος "boat" and κεφαλή "head") is the most frequent form of craniosynostosis (60% of all craniosynostosis with a male predilection, 3:1). Scaphocephaly is a premature suture of the sagittal suture producing deformation of the skull with an increase in the anteroposterior axis (with a CI lower than 75%). The premature closure of the sagittal suture prevents the skull from growing in the latero-lateral axis but can grow anteroposteriorly, producing a narrow and elongated skull. In this case, there is rarely hydrocephalus or a decrease in the intelligence quotient (IQ) (Fig. 6).

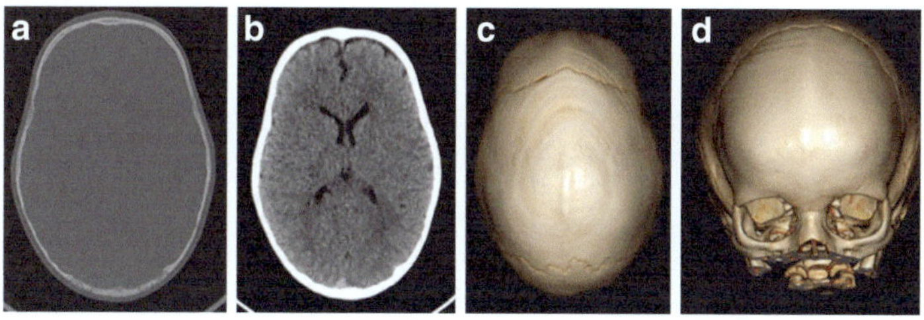

FIGURE 6 Head CT scan axial reconstructions (**a** and **b**) and 3D VRT (**c** and **d**) in a 14-month-old male with scaphocephaly in premature sagittal suture closure. Note the normal aspect of the ventricular system

Trigonocephaly

Trigonocephaly (from the Greek word τρίγωνο, "triangle") is defined by premature closure of the metopic suture resulting in an angle in the forehead and a triangle-shaped skull and accounts for 10% of all craniosynostosis. Due to these frontal bone modifications, the eyes are closer (hypotelorism), and the face is narrow (Fig. 7).

Plagiocephaly

Unilateral closure of the coronal or the lambdoid suture results in plagiocephaly (from the Greek πλάγιος, "oblique" and κεφαλή, "head") and is associated with an antero- or posterolateral, respectively, deformation of the skull, occurs in 1 to 10,000 live births. Plagiocephaly can also be non-synostotic due to a prolonged pre- or postnatal vicious position of the head (Fig. 8).

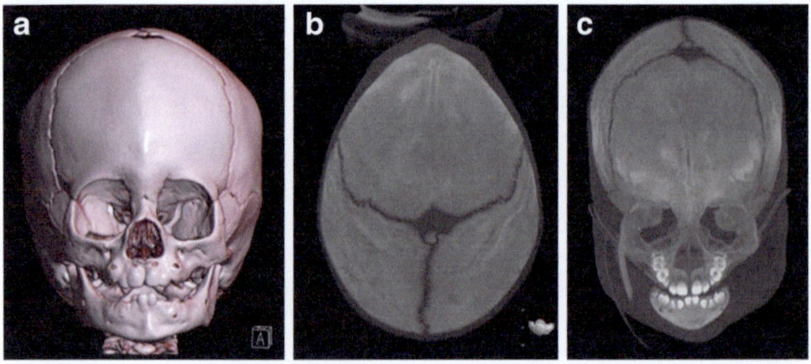

FIGURE 7 (**a**) CT scan 3D VRT, (**b**) axial oblique maximum intensity projection (MIP) 50 mm, and (**c**) coronal MIP 50 mm reconstruction. Trigonocephaly in a 6-month-old girl (premature closure of the metopic suture) leading to a triangle-shaped forehead and a narrow and elongated skull

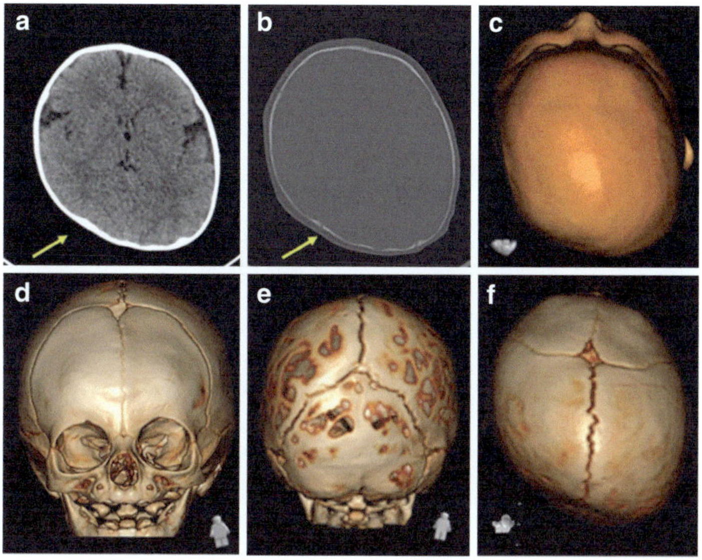

FIGURE 8 Head CT scan in a 4-month-old female girl with non-synostotic plagiocephaly (yellow arrow). (**a**) Axial plane in soft tissue, (**b**) in an axial plane in bony reconstruction, and (**c**–**f**) 3D VRT reconstructions

Brachycephaly

When the coronal or the lambdoid sutures close prematurely, the anteroposterior axis of the skull is reduced along with a facial elevation providing brachycephaly (from the Greek βραχύς "short" and κεφαλή "head") with a CI greater than 80%.

Oxycephaly (Acrocephaly)

The early closure of all the sutures results in oxycephaly (from the Greek οξύς, "sharp", "pointed head"), which causes,

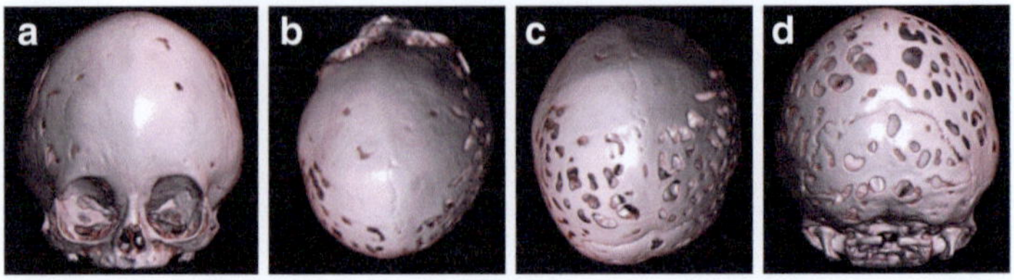

FIGURE 9 3D VRT reconstructions in a head CT in an 8-month-old boy with multi-sutural premature closure (oxycephaly) (**a**) frontal view, (**b**) superior view, (**c**) postero superior view, (**d**) posterior view. Note the thinning of the skull in D

on the one hand, reduced skull growth (microcephaly) and, on the other hand, increased intracranial pressure as well as an increased risk of mental retardation (Fig. 9). Increased intracranial pressure can result in hydrocephalus, evaluated by the Evans index. The Evans index is a ratio between the maximal width of the frontal horns of the lateral ventricles and the biparietal diameter on an axial plane on CT or MRI (Fig. 10). The normal Evans index is less than 30%.

Acrocephaly is often seen in Crouzon or Apert syndrome.

Syndromic Craniosynostosis

The most characteristics findings in syndromic craniosynostosis are microcephaly, hypertelorism, exorbitism, midface hypoplasia, pancraniosynostis and skull deformation. The most frequent syndromic craniosynostosis are the Apert, the Crouzon and the Pfeiffer syndromes (Fig. 11).

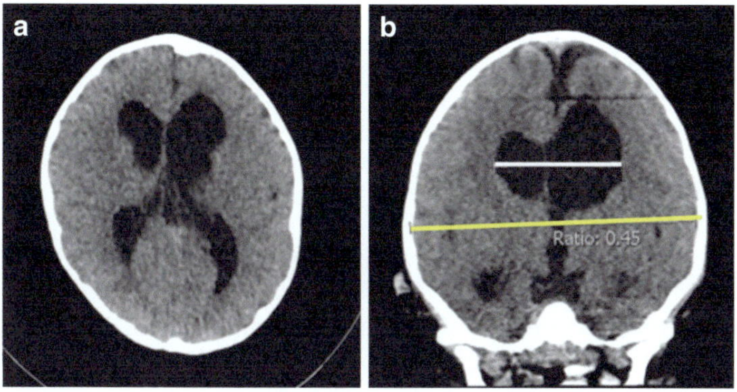

FIGURE 10 Head CT scan, (**a**) axial plane, (**b**) coronal plane, in the same 8-month-old boy with multi-sutural premature closure (oxycephaly) and hydrocephalus. Evans's index is 0.45. The normal Evan's index is less than 0.30 (30%)

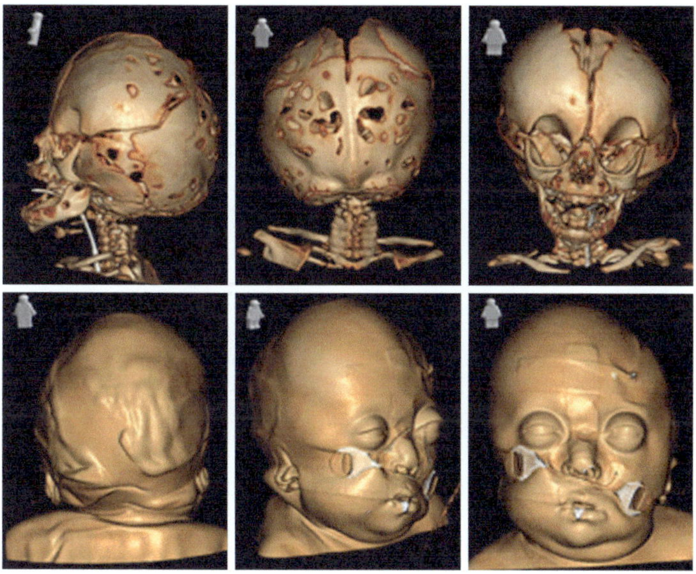

FIGURE 11 3D VRT reconstruction of a head CT scan in a 1-month-old girl with Pfeiffer syndrome presenting with exorbitism and craniosynostosis

Craniocervical Junction

The craniocervical junction is a complex anatomical area that contains the central nervous system (the brain stem and the spinal cord), vascular structures, bones (Fig. 12) and ligaments. Many parameters in the anatomy of the craniocervical junction in children are immature, inducing a hypermobile craniocervical junction because of ligament hyperlaxity in the cervical spine. The stability of the craniocervical junction is paramount to support the weight of a child's head. At birth, the brain is typically 25% of its adult size, although the body weight of the newborn is only about 5% of adult weight [15].

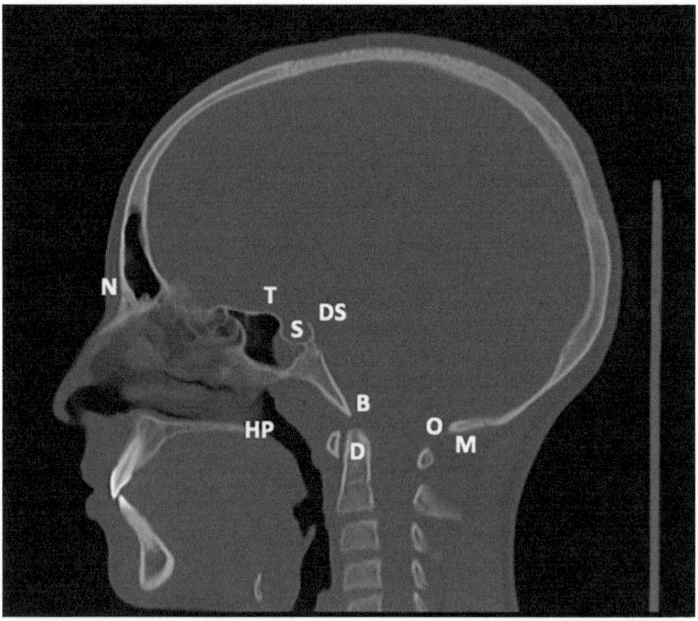

FIGURE 12 *N*: nasion, *T*: tuberculum sellae, *S*: sella turcica, *DS*: dorsum sellae, *B*: basion, *D*: dens, *HP*: hard palate, *O*: opisthion, *M*: most caudal point of the cranium

Skull Base Craniometry

Skull base craniometry in the assessment of craniocervical junction malformations is paramount (Fig. 13):

- McRae's line connects the anterior and the posterior margins of the foramen magnum (basion to the opisthion). The tip of the odontoid process projects 5 mm above McRae's line.
- Chamberlain's line is a line joining the posterior edge of the hard palate to the opisthion. The tip of the odontoid process may project above this line up to 1 mm (±6.6 mm).
- McGregor developed a modified Chamberlain's line for when the opisthion is not well detected on lateral radiograph. This line connects the hard palate and the most caudal part of the occipital curve. The tip of the odontoid process usually projects not more than 5 mm above the McGregor line.
- Wackenheim's line (also known as the basilar line or clival line) draws the posterior aspect of the clivus and falls tangential to the posterior aspect of the odontoid process. In the case of basilar invagination, the odontoid process crosses this line.

The following angles in the craniocervical junction craniometry are the most used for the imaging workup of the craniocervical junction (Fig. 14):

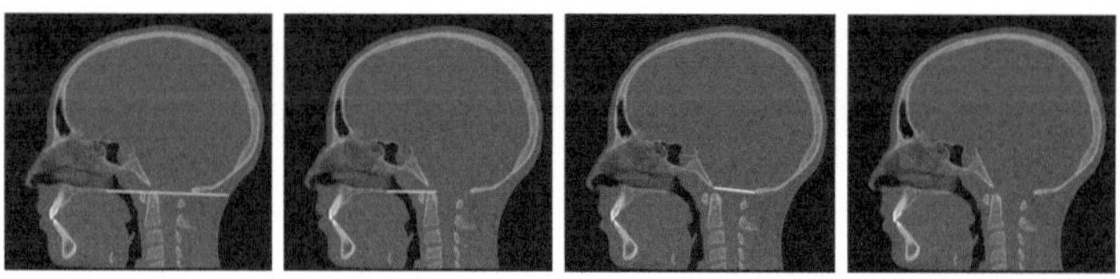

FIGURE 13 Green line, Mc Gregor line; blue line, Chamberlain's line; yellow line, McRae's line; pink line: Wackenheim's clivus canal line

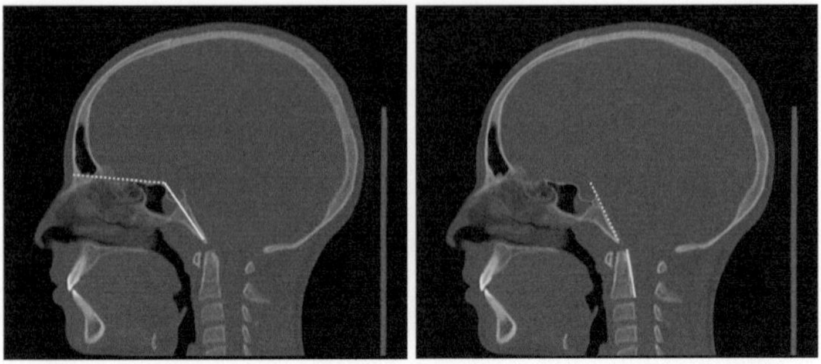

FIGURE 14 Welcher angle (dotted and bold white lines) and craniovertebral angle (dotted and bold yellow lines) in a 14-year-old boy

- The Welcher basal angle is measured at the intersection of the line connecting the nasion to the tuberculum sellae and the line connecting the tuberculum sellae to the basion (normal values between 122 and 132°). When abnormal, the Welcher angle allows the diagnosis of platybasia (>143°) and basilar kyphosis (<125°).
- The craniovertebral angle is formed by the tangent line at the clivus and the tangent line at the odontoid process (150–180°).

Odontoid Process

The odontoid process belongs to the second cervical vertebra (or axis) and has a complex embryological development. The ossification centre of the apex of the odontoid process appears between the age of 3 and 6 years and fuses at the age of 12 years [16]. The fusion of the odontoid process with the C2 body fuses between 3 and 6 years old. The fusion line in between is called subdental synchondrosis and can be detected until 11 years (not to be mistaken with a fracture). The posterior arches of the axis fuse at 2–3 years and with the body of the odontoid process at 3–6 years [16].

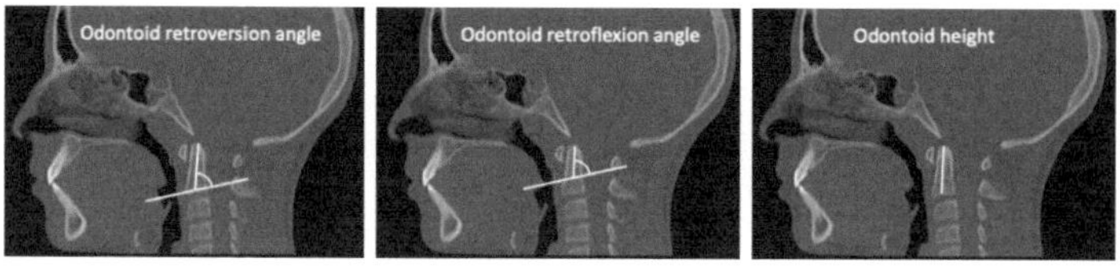

FIGURE 15 Sagittal CT scan MPR with the odontoid retroversion angle, the odontoid retroflexion angle and the odontoid process height

The odontoid process is shorter and more anteriorly inclined in children than adults. The odontoid retroversion angle in children is 71.9 ± 5.3°, the odontoid retroflexion angle in children is between 79.3 ± 4.9°, and the range of the odontoid process height in children is 17–27 mm (Fig. 15) [17].

The distance between the basion and the tip of the odontoid process should be equal to or less than 12 mm [16]. The atlodens interval (ADI) is the distance between the anterior aspect of the odontoid process and the posterior aspect of the first cervical vertebra and should be less than 5 mm in children [16]. An atlodens interval wider than 5 mm suggests a ligament disruption and an unstable posttraumatic lesion [16].

Basilar Invagination (Congenital): Atlantoaxial Impaction

Basilar invagination is a congenital upward displacement of vertebral elements into a normal foramen magnum with normal bone and is present when the tip of the dens is >2.5 mm above Chamberlain's line [18]. For the cases in which the opisthion cannot be identified on plain radiographs, McGregor developed a modification of Chamberlain's line. The tip of the odontoid process usually projects not more than 5 mm above the McGregor line.

Basilar Impression (Acquired)

Basilar impression (acquired) is an upward displacement of the dens due to an abnormal softening of bones at the base of the skull. Basilar impression is often associated with osteogenesis imperfecta [19].

Chiari I (Arnold-Chiari) Malformation

Chiari I malformation is defined by the downward displacement of the cerebellar tonsils through the foramen magnum into the spinal canal (Fig. 16). Posterior angulation of the odontoid process is associated with Chiari I malformation [20]. A mild tonsillar ectopia is defined when the tonsillar herniation is less than 3–5 mm. The true Chiari I malformation is defined as a tonsillar herniation of more than 3–5 mm below McRae's line. The Chiari I malformation is frequently associated with hydro (syringo) myelia and hydrocephalus, and a complete imaging workup of the entire neuraxis is mandatory.

Up to one third (2–38%) of Chiari I malformation is associated with basilar invagination, and in that case, the cranio-

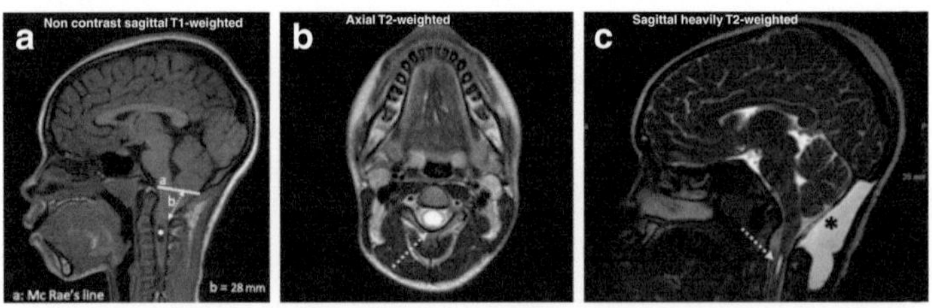

FIGURE 16 Arnold-Chiari I malformation in a 14-year-old girl showing in (**a**, **b**) the preoperative MRI showing descent of the cerebellum of 28 mm and a syrinx (asterisk in **a** and yellow dotted arrow in **b**). The postoperative MRI on (**c**) shows a less pointed cerebellum located in the posterior fossa and is associated with a pseudo-meningocele (black asterisk), secondary to the surgical management. The syrinx is also visible (yellow dotted arrow)

cervical junction is unstable [21]. When patients with Chiari I malformation and craniocervical junction instability complain of debilitating occipital headaches, neck pain, myelopathy, hyperreflexia or even dysphagia [21], surgical management is the therapeutical option.

References

1. Jin SW, Sim KB, Kim SD. Development and growth of the normal cranial vault: an embryologic review. J Korean Neurosurg Soc. 2016;59(3):192.
2. Opperman LA. Cranial sutures as intramembranous bone growth sites. Dev Dyn. 2000;219(4):472–85.
3. Mitchell LA, Kitley CA, Armitage TL, Krasnokutsky MV, Rooks VJ. Normal sagittal and coronal suture widths by using CT imaging. Am J Neuroradiol. 2011;32(10):1801–5.
4. Nayak SR, Krishnamurthy A, Madhan Kumar SJ, Prabhu LV, Jiji PJ, Pai MM, et al. The mendosal suture of the occipital bone: occurrence in Indian population, embryology and clinical significance. Surg Radiol Anat. 2007;29(4):329–32.
5. Idriz S, Patel JH, Ameli Renani S, Allan R, Vlahos I. CT of normal developmental and variant anatomy of the pediatric skull: distinguishing trauma from normality. Radiographics. 2015;35(5):1585–601.
6. Popich GA, Smith DW. Fontanels: range of normal size. J Pediatr. 1972;80(5):749–52.
7. D'Antoni AV, Donaldson OI, Schmidt C, Macchi V, De Caro R, Oskouian RJ, et al. A comprehensive review of the anterior Fontanelle: embryology, anatomy, and clinical considerations. Childs Nerv Syst. 2017;33(6):909–14.
8. Madeline LA, Elster AD. Suture closure in the human chondrocranium: CT assessment. Radiology. 1995;196(3):747–56.
9. Raybaud C. In: Barkovich AJ, editor. Pediatric neuroimaging. 5th ed. Philadelphia, PA: Wolters Kluwer/Lippincott Williams & Wilkins; 2012. p. 1125.
10. Chumas PD, Cinalli G, Arnaud E, Marchac D, Renier D. Classification of previously unclassified cases of craniosynostosis. J Neurosurg. 1997;86(2):177–81.
11. Hadlock F, Deter R, Carpenter R, Park S. Estimating fetal age: effect of head shape on BPD. Am J Roentgenol. 1981;137(1):83–5.

12. Simanovsky N, Hiller N, Koplewitz B, Rozovsky K. Effectiveness of ultrasonographic evaluation of the cranial sutures in children with suspected craniosynostosis. Eur Radiol. 2009;19(3):687–92.
13. Chatterjee JS, Mahmoud M, Karthikeyan S, Duncan C, Dover MS, Nishikawa H. Referral pattern and surgical outcome of sagittal synostosis. J Plast Reconstr Aesthet Surg. 2009;62(2):211–5.
14. Mathijssen IMJ. Guideline for care of patients with the diagnoses of craniosynostosis: working group on craniosynostosis. J Craniofac Surg. 2015;26(6):1735–807.
15. Stuart HC, Stevenson SS. Physical growth and development. In: Mitchell-Nelson, editor. Textbook of pediatrics. 5th ed. Philadelphia: American Psychological Association; 1950.
16. Lustrin ES, Karakas SP, Ortiz AO, Cinnamon J, Castillo M, Vaheesan K, et al. Pediatric cervical spine: normal anatomy, variants, and trauma. Radiographics. 2003;23(3):539–60.
17. Khaleel ZL, Besachio DA, Bisson EF, Shah LM. Estimation of odontoid process posterior inclination, odontoid height, and pB–C2 line in the adult population: clinical article. J Neurosurg Spine. 2014;20(2):172–7.
18. Baysal B, Eser MB, Sorkun M. Radiological approach to basilar invagination type B: reliability and accuracy. J Neuroradiol. 2022;49(1):33–40.
19. Pinter NK, McVige J, Mechtler L. Basilar invagination, basilar impression, and platybasia: clinical and imaging aspects. Curr Pain Headache Rep. 2016;20(8):49.
20. Lang J, Lang J. Clinical anatomy of the cervical spine. Stuttgart, New York: Thieme; 1993. p. 192.
21. Goldstein HE, Anderson RCE. Craniovertebral junction instability in the setting of Chiari I malformation. Neurosurg Clin N Am. 2015;26(4):561–9.

Spine

Mandip K. Heir, Amit Shah, and Winston J. Rennie

Spine

When the paediatric spine develops, important morphological and biomechanical changes occur, during the synchronised growth of the vertebral bodies, posterior arches, spinal cord and roots [1].

Vertebrae formed as somites derived from paraxial mesoderm at 3 weeks of gestational age begin to surround the neural tube and notochord, forming a sclerotome. These sclerotome cells on either side of the cord migrate around the cord merging together at 4 weeks of gestational age. Segmentation of these sclerotomes forms the vertebral bodies [2].

M. K. Heir (✉)
Leicester Royal Infirmary, Infirmary Square, Leicester, UK
e-mail: mandip.heir@uhl-tr.nhs.uk

A. Shah
Leicester Royal Infirmary, Infirmary Square, Leicester, UK
e-mail: amit.shah2@nhs.net

W. J. Rennie
Leicester Royal Infirmary, Infirmary Square, Leicester, UK

Loughborough University, Loughborough, UK
e-mail: winston.rennie@uhl-tr.nhs.uk

P. Simoni, M. P. Aparisi Gómez (eds.), *Essential Measurements in Pediatric Musculoskeletal Imaging*,
https://doi.org/10.1007/978-3-031-17735-4_3

Chondrogenesis and then endochondral ossification of the vertebral bodies start at 40–60 days gestational age, with ossification continuing up to 25 years of age [3]. The three primary ossification centres are the vertebral body and bilateral neural ossification centres forming a neurocentral synchondrosis, contributing to vertebral body, spinal canal and posterior element development. Five secondary ossification centres include the superior and inferior surfaces of the vertebral body, transverse process tips and spinous process tip.

At term the oval ossified nucleus of the vertebral body is small relative to the large cartilaginous endplates, with unfused neurocentral synchondrosis. The neurocentral synchondrosis closes at different ages within the cervical, thoracic and lumbar spine, up to the age of 17 years [4]. As the ossification of the vertebral bodies and posterior elements completes, the spinal canal diameter reduces.

Cervical spine curvature is present in utero, secondary to head weight and uterine constraints [5]. The primary curves of the spine at birth are the thoracic and sacral curves. Biomechanical changes when able to hold the head and when able to weightbear result in the normal cervical and lumbar lordosis curvatures of the spine [2]. By the age of 10 years, the spinal curvature is similar to an adult, although absence of cervical lordosis can be seen up to the age of 16 years [6].

Cervical Spine

Basilar Invagination/Impression

Basilar impression is the upward displacement of the vertebral elements with normal bone, into a normal foramen magnum. Basilar invagination is similar upward displacement due to pathology of the bones [7]:

- Chamberlain line (Fig. 1): Line drawn from posterior margin of the hard palate to opisthion (posterior margin of the foramen magnum). Tip of odontoid process should normally be <2.5 mm above this line. If the odontoid process

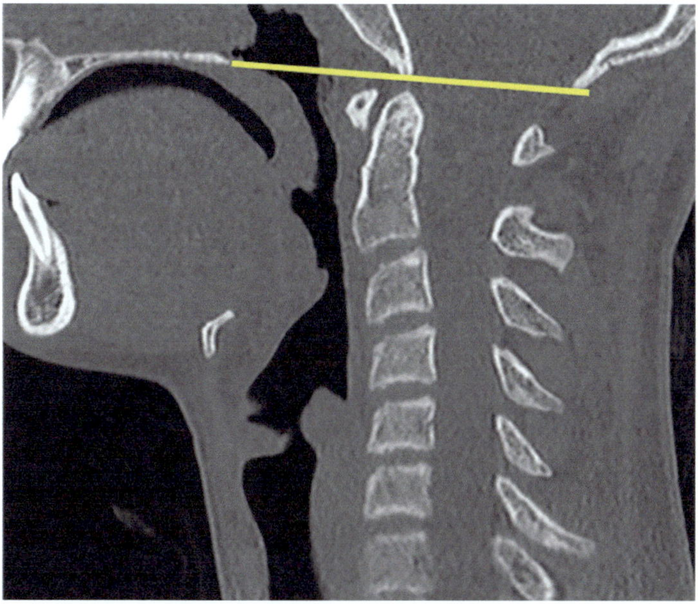

FIGURE 1 A sagittal CT image demonstrating the Chamberlain line

tip is >2.5 mm above the line, there is basilar invagination [8]. However, using this criterion alone to diagnose basilar invagination may lead to high false positives [9].

- Clivodens angle (Fig. 2): Angle formed when line drawn along long axis of clivus and long axis of dens. A value of <125° suggests basilar invagination [9].

Atlanto-Occipital Junction

- Basion-dens interval in assessing atlanto-occipital dislocation (Fig. 3): Distance between the basion and the odontoid process of C2 should be 12 mm or less [6]. This measurement should be used cautiously in children as the odontoid height increases with age in normal development. Under 9 years of age, the odontoid is shorter than the level of the anterior arch of C1 height [10].

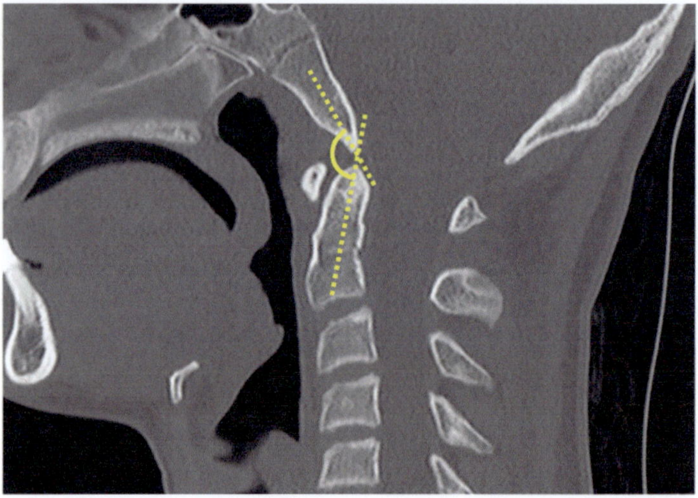

FIGURE 2 A sagittal CT image demonstrating the Clivodens angle

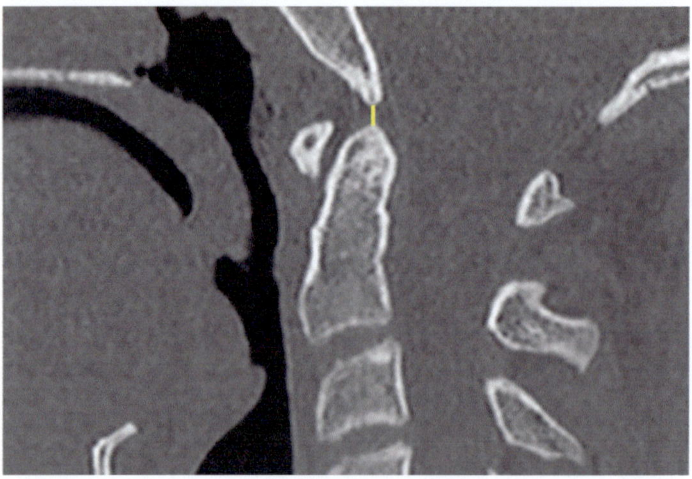

FIGURE 3 A sagittal CT image demonstrating the basion-dens interval

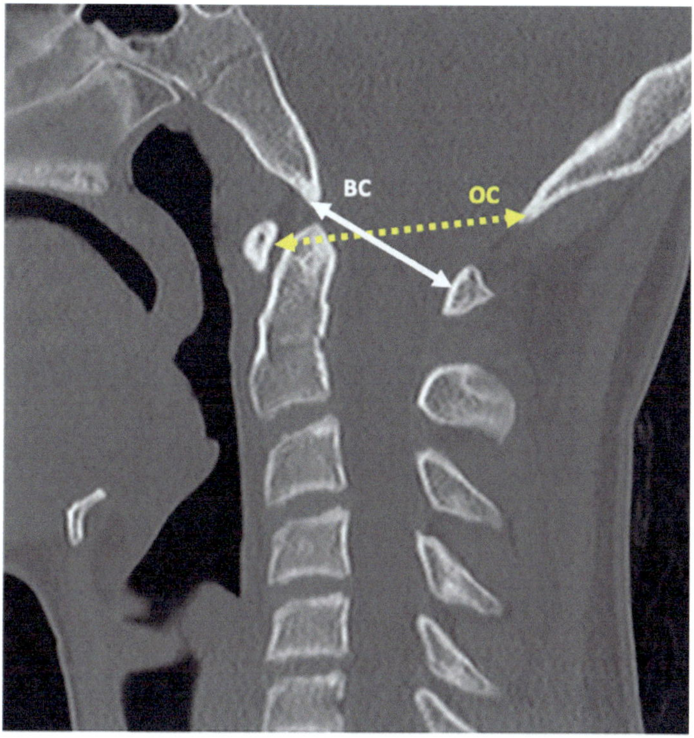

FIGURE 4 A sagittal CT image demonstrating the lines drawn to calculate Powers ratio (BC/OC). *BC:* basion to posterior C1 (in white) and *OC:* ophistion to anterior C1 (in dotted yellow)

- Powers ratio to detect subluxation/dislocation (Fig. 4): Distance from the tip of the basion to the posterior arch of C1 (BC) divided by the distance from the opisthion to the anterior arch of C1 (OC). A Powers ratio (BC/OC) of less than 1 is considered standard on radiographs. On CT, a ratio of less than 0.9 (midline sagittal plane) is considered standard. A Powers ratio (BC/OC) of more than 1 on flexion and extension views is diagnostic of anterior atlanto-occipital instability [11].

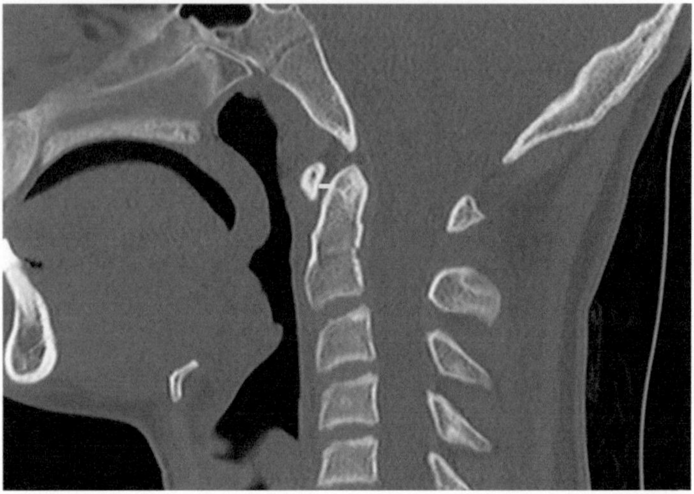

FIGURE 5 A sagittal CT image demonstrating the atlanto-dens interval

Atlanto-Dens Interval (ADI)

This is an important measurement when assessing atlanto-axial subluxation. The ADI is measured between the posteroinferior margin of the anterior arch of the atlas and the anterior surface of the odontoid process (Fig. 5). Extension/flexion of the cervical spine during positioning can affect ADI measurement; hence, ADI should be measured in neutral position [12]. Normal values in neutral position are <4 mm in children <9 years of age and <3 mm in children >9 years age [13].

Posterior Atlanto-Dens Relationship

If a posterior ligamentous injury is suspected on lateral X-rays performed in flexion, the posterior atlanto-dens relationship can be assessed. The ratio between the posterior arch

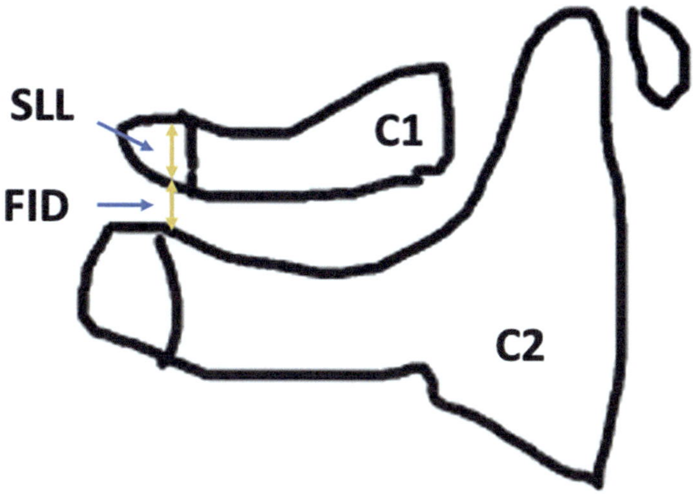

FIGURE 6 A diagram demonstrating the spinolaminar line (SLL) and flexion interspinous distance (FID)

of C1 at the spinolaminar line (SLL) and the interspinous distance between C1 and C2 (FID) in flexion is calculated (Fig. 6). FID/SLL >2 suggests a posterior ligamentous injury in all ages [14].

Posterior Cervical Line/Posterior Line of Swischuk

Anterior displacement of C2 on C3 has been observed in children up to the age of 7 years [15]. The posterior cervical (Swischuk) line (Fig. 7) helps differentiate physiological displacement/pseudosubluxation from pathological subluxation. The posterior cervical/Swischuk line is drawn through the anterior cortex of the posterior arches of C1–C3.

In pathological subluxation, the line will miss the posterior arch of C2 by more than 2 mm [15] (Fig. 8).

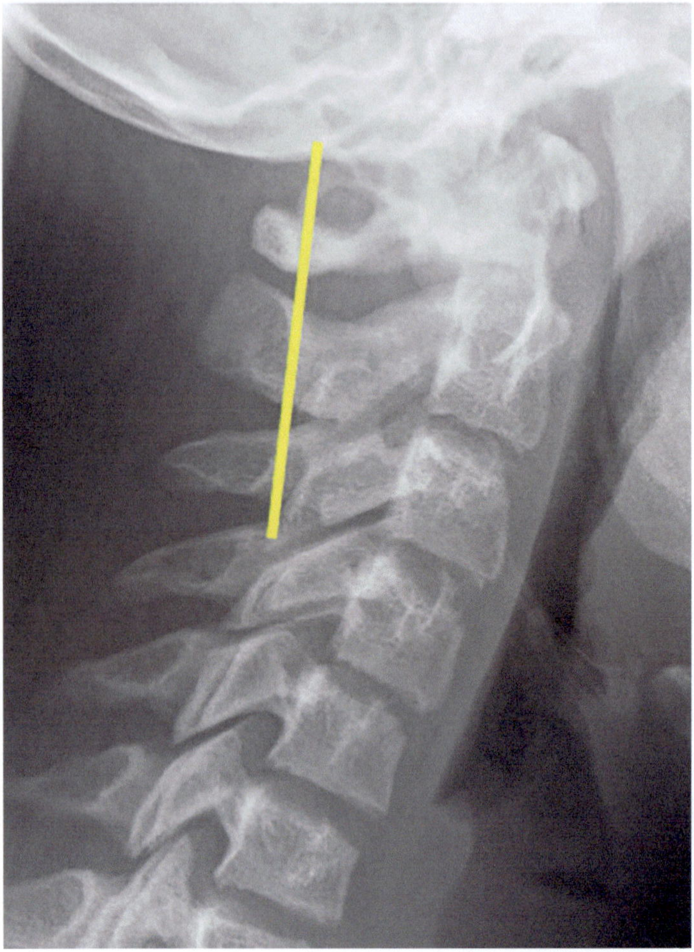

FIGURE 7 A lateral X-ray demonstrating the posterior cervical line/ posterior line of Swischuk

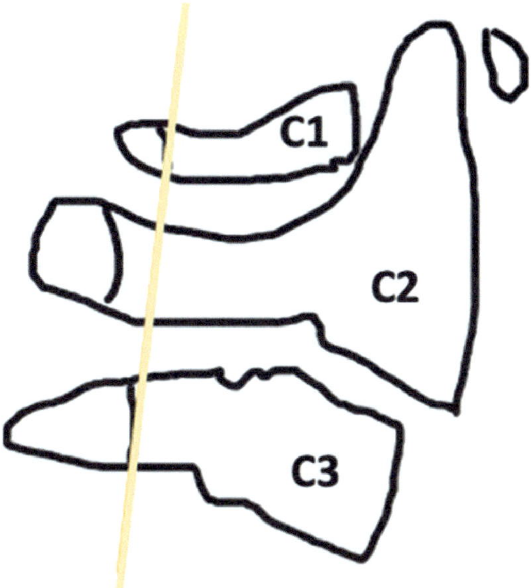

FIGURE 8 A diagram demonstrating pathological subluxation of C2 in relation to C3

Prevertebral Soft Tissue Assessment

- The prevertebral soft tissue thickness aids in the detection of cervical spine injuries. Thickness can be measured on both lateral cervical spine X-ray and sagittal CT, at C2 and C6 levels (Fig. 9), given the reduced variability in the measurements at these levels (Table 1).

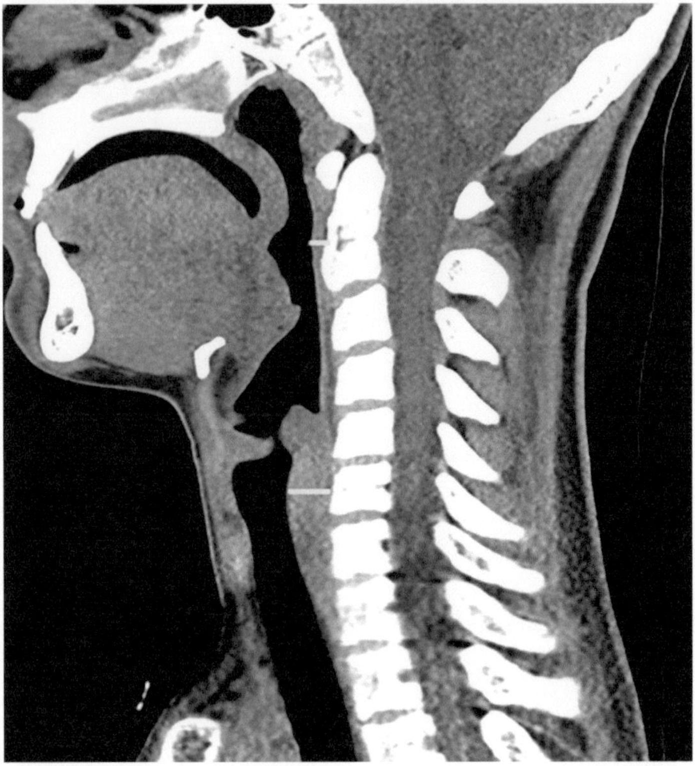

FIGURE 9 A sagittal CT image demonstrating the prevertebral soft tissue thickness at C2 and C6 vertebral levels

TABLE 1 Mean values of prevertebral soft tissue thickness at C2 and C6 levels, measured on MDCT [16]

Age (years)	Mean prevertebral soft tissue thickness at C2 (mm) mean ± SD	Mean prevertebral soft tissue thickness at C6 (mm) mean ± SD
0–2	5.0 ± 1.3	6.3 ± 1.4
3–6	5.0 ± 1.7	7.5 ± 1.2
7–10	4.6 ± 1.1	9.1 ± 1.5
11–15	4.6 ± 1.1	10.9 ± 1.8
18 years plus	3.7 ± 1.2	13.0 ± 2.6

Spinal Canal Size

After the age of 4 years, only minimal growth of the spinal canal diameter occurs, increasing on average 3.2 mm at C2 and 2.6 mm at C7 in males and 2.8 mm and 2.0 mm in females, respectively (Table 2) [17].

Vertebral Body Height

Cervical vertebral body height increases with age and growth, as well as changing from an oval morphology to rectangular (Table 3).

TABLE 2 Cervical spine canal AP dimension at C2 and C7 (modified from [17])

	Male		**Female**	
Age (years)	**C2 diameter (mm) mean ± SD**	**C7 diameter (mm) mean ± SD**	**C2 diameter (mm) mean ± SD**	**C7 diameter (mm) mean ± SD**
1	14.41 ± 1.23	13.35 ± 1.35	13.53 ± 1.28	12.56 ± 0.89
4	16.23 ± 1.05	14.91 ± 0.94	15.30 ± 1.59	14.56 ± 0.90
9	16.99 ± 1.21	15.06 ± 1.18	16.12 ± 1.00	14.12 ± 0.85
15	15.70 ± 1.43	14.53 ± 1.17	15.61 ± 1.67	14.15 ± 1.06

TABLE 3 Cervical body height at C3 and C5 (modified from [18])

	Male		**Female**	
Age (years)	**C3 vertebral body height (mm) mean ± SD**	**C5 vertebral body height (mm) mean ± SD**	**C3 vertebral body height (mm) mean ± SD**	**C5 vertebral body height (mm) mean ± SD**
0–5	5.52 ± 1.18	5.47 ± 1.19	5.84 ± 1.18	5.74 ± 1.12
5–10	7.82 ± 1.29	7.53 ± 0.99	8.09 ± 1.20	7.69 ± 1.10
10–15	11.51 ± 2.45	10.51 ± 2.10	11.56 ± 2.69	10.79 ± 2.16

Thoracolumbar Spine

Thoracic Kyphosis

- The spine has characteristic alignment in the coronal and sagittal planes. In the sagittal plane, the spine is lordotic in the cervical and lumbar regions and kyphotic in the thoracic region.
- The thoracic kyphosis angle increases with age and the increase is greater in females than in males.
- Kyphosis is a marked curvature of the spine in the sagittal plane, with a posterior convexity.
- According to the Scoliosis Research Society classification system, the curvature in the sagittal plane is normally smooth and comprised between 20° and 45°.

Modified Cobb Angle

- The upper (commonly T4/5) and lower (commonly T12) vertebral bodies defining the curve are selected and lines are drawn, extending along the superior border of the upper end vertebra as well as along the inferior border of the lower end vertebra. Perpendicular lines are drawn from these and the angle is measured at the intersection (most modern PACS systems will have angle tools that measure directly as in Fig. 10).

Sagittal Balance

- Essential for the spine body to maintain equilibrium. Alterations affect forces and energy required to maintain a horizontal gaze in the upright position.
- Sagittal balance is evaluated by measuring the distance between the posterosuperior aspect of the S1 vertebral body and the plumb line.

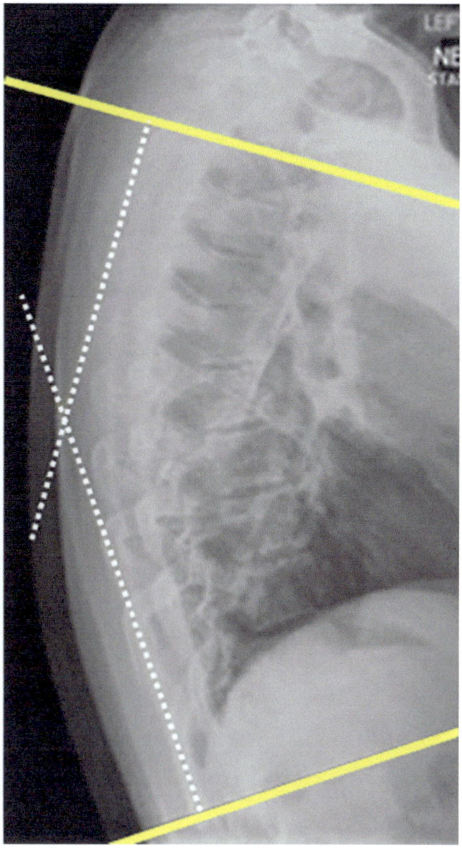

FIGURE 10 A lateral X-ray demonstrating modified Cobb angle measurement

C7 Plumb Line

- The plumb line is a vertical line drawn downwards from the centre of the C7 vertebral body, parallel to the lateral edges of the radiograph (Fig. 11).
- This line should pass through the superior endplate of S1, ± 2 cm of the posterosuperior corner of the S1 vertebral body [19, 20].

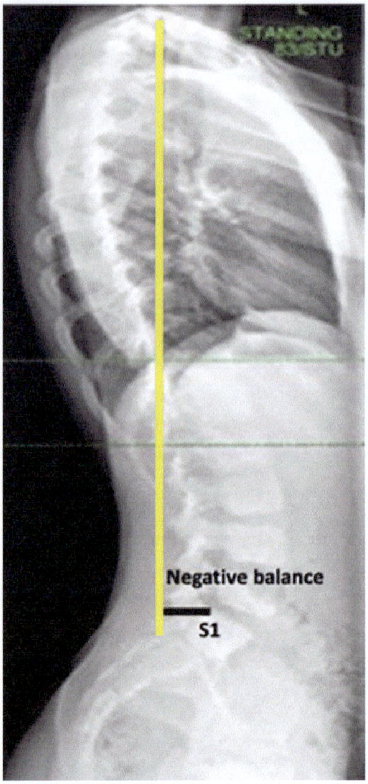

FIGURE 11 A lateral X-ray demonstrating the C7 plumb line

- The position of this line is can be positive, neutral or negative:
  - Positive balance: the plumb line passes more than 2 cm in front of the posterosuperior corner of the S1 vertebral body.
  - Neutral balance: the plumb line passes within 2 cm of the posterosuperior corner of the S1 vertebral body.
  - Negative balance: the plumb line passes more than 2 cm behind the posterosuperior corner of the S1 vertebral body.

Scoliosis

- Represents the presence of one or more lateral curves of the vertebral column in the coronal plane.

- Scoliosis is defined as a lateral spinal curvature with a Cobb angle of >10°.
- The Scoliosis Research Society classifies paediatric scoliosis as [21]:
  - Infantile 0–3.
  - Juvenile 4–10.
  - Adolescent 11–18.

Infantile Idiopathic Scoliosis

- 1.5× more frequent in boys than girls.
- 76% of cases scoliosis is left convex.
- Many infants with infantile idiopathic scoliosis are healthy and normal and simply have a small curvature of the spine. In some patients, however, there is an increased association with hip dysplasia, mental retardation and congenital heart disease.
- Many infantile curves will resolve without treatment.

Juvenile Idiopathic Scoliosis

- 10–15% of all idiopathic scoliosis in children.
- Early years, boys are affected slightly more than girls and the curve is often left-sided.
- Later years, predominance of girls and right-sided curves.
- As a rule of thumb, about 20% of children who are younger than 10 and who have a curve greater than 20° will have an underlying spinal condition (particularly an Arnold-Chiari malformation).
- Juvenile curves that reach 25–30° tend to continue to worsen without treatment.

Cobb Angle

- Lines are drawn along the endplates of the *terminale vertebrae*, and the angle between the two lines, where they intersect, is measured.
- The *cephalad* and *caudal terminale vertebra* are those vertebrae whose endplates are most tilted towards each other

(most modern PACS systems will have angle tools that measure directly as in Fig. 12).

- Mild 10–15°.
- Moderate 20–40°.
- Severe >40°.

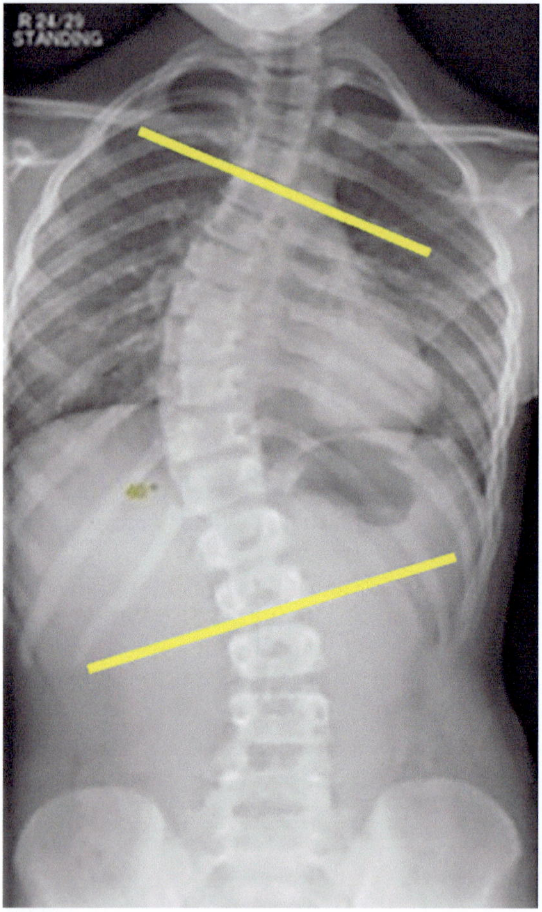

FIGURE 12 An anteroposterior X-ray demonstrating the Cobb angle

Coronal Balance

- Coronal balance is evaluated by measuring the distance between the central sacral vertical line (CSVL) and the plumb line.
- It measures whether or not the upper spine is located over the midline (normal) or off to one side.
- The CSVL is a vertical line that is drawn perpendicular to an imaginary tangential line drawn across the top of the iliac crests on radiographs. It bisects the sacrum.
- The plumb line is a vertical line drawn downwards from the centre of the C7 vertebral body, parallel to the lateral edges of the radiograph.
- The horizontal distance between this plumb line and the CSVL is measured (Fig. 13).
- The position of this line can then termed positive, neutral or negative, depending on distance and direction from the midline:
  - Positive balance: the plumb line passes to the right of the midline, by >2 cm.
  - Neutral balance: the plumb line passes within 2 cm of the midline.
  - Negative balance: the plumb line passes to the left of the midline, by >2 cm.

Lumbar Spinal Canal Dimensions

- Anteroposterior spinal canal development is fully complete by 5 years of age, while transverse spinal canal diameter increases until 15–17 years [22, 23].
- Considerable variation in the developmental size of the normal lumbar spinal canal exists within and between populations.
- The sagittal diameter is the shortest midline perpendicular distance from the vertebral body to the inner surface of the neural arch (Table 4) [24].

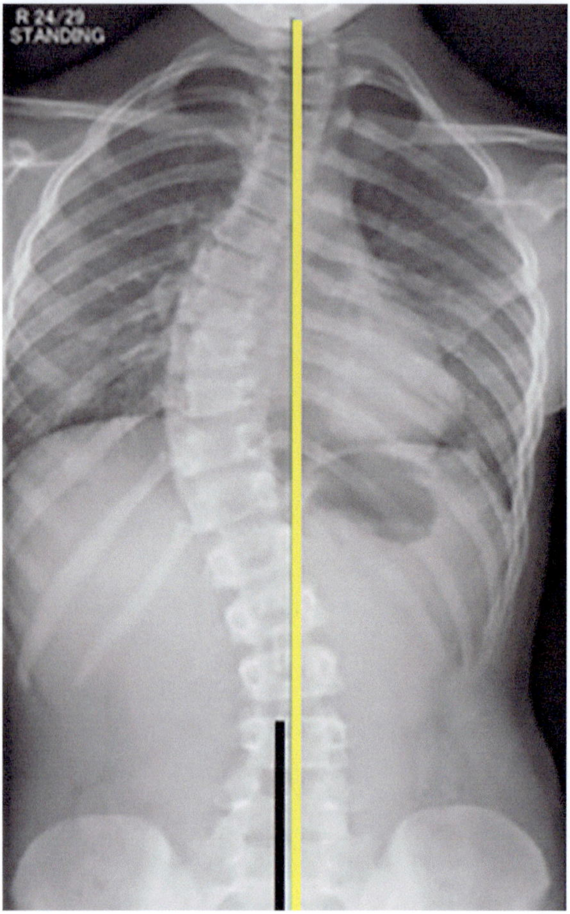

FIGURE 13 An anteroposterior X-ray demonstrating coronal balance (short black line is the CSVL and yellow line is the plumb line)

TABLE 4 Radiographic spinal canal dimensions [24]

	Spinal canal dimensions (mm) minimum-maximum				
Age (years)	**L1**	**L2**	**L3**	**L4**	**L5**
3–5	16–24	16–24	15–22	15–22	15–22
6–8	15–25	15–25	14–24	14–24	14–24
9–10	16–24	16–24	15–23	15–23	15–23
11–12	15–26	14–25	14–24	14–24	15–25
13–14	17–24	17–23	16–22	13–28	13–28
15–16	16–24	16–24	15–23	15–23	15–23
17–18	16–28	16–28	16–28	16–28	16–28

- Knirsch et al. measured the sagittal diameters of the lumbar spine (vertebral body and dural sac) on MRI in 75 healthy children (32 boys, 43 girls) between 6 years and 17 years of age (Table 5).
- Measurements are made perpendicular to the long axis of the vertebral body and the dural sac (Fig. 14). The dural sac dimension (DSD) was measured as the longest distance between the posterior border of the vertebral body and the anterior border of the spinous process.

Table 5 MRI spinal canal dimensions in mm [25]

Age (years)	MRI spinal canal dimensions (mm) mean ± SD					
	L1	**L2**	**L3**	**L4**	**L5**	**S1**
6–8	16.1 ± 1.8	15.6 ± 1.5	14.5 ± 1.4	14.1 ± 1.3	15.1 ± 2.1	13.7 ± 1.7
9–11	17.1 ± 1.3	16.1 ± 1.1	15.6 ± 1.5	15.7 ± 1.9	15.9 ± 1.2	14.6 ± 2.0
12–14	17.7 ± 1.9	16.7 ± 1.8	16.2 ± 1.7	16.7 ± 1.9	16.9 ± 2.4	14.7 ± 2.9
15–17	17.6 ± 1.8	16.4 ± 1.8	15.5 ± 1.5	16.4 ± 1.6	17.4 ± 2.3	15.0 ± 2.5

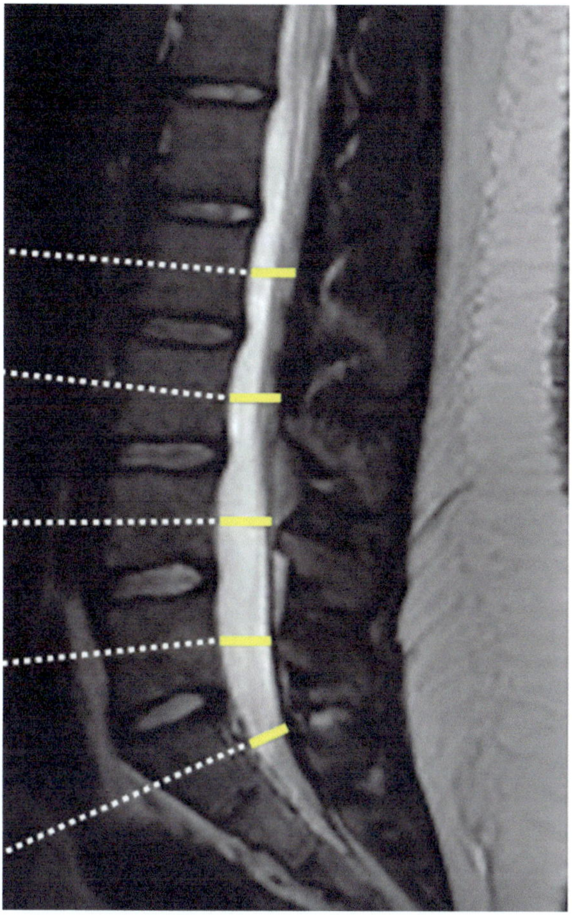

Figure 14 A sagittal T2 MR image demonstrating spinal canal dimension measurements

References

1. Raimondi AJ, Choux M, Di Rocco C. The paediatric spine I: development and the Dysraphic state. New York: Springer-Verlag; 1989. p. 39–40. (A DiMeglio and F Bonnel. Chapter 3 Growth of the spine pages 39-40).

2. Aparisi Gomez MP, Watkin S, Perry D, et al. Anatomical considerations of embryology and development of the musculoskeletal system: basic notions for musculoskeletal radiologists. Semin Musculoskelet Radiol. 2021;25:3–21. https://doi.org/10.1055/s-0041-1723005.
3. Colafati GS, Marrazzo A, Marco C, et al. The paediatric spine. Semin Musculoskelet Radiol. 2021;25:137–54. https://doi.org/10.1055/s-0041-1727095.
4. Blakemore L, Schwend R, Akbarnia BA, Dumas M, Schmidt J. Growth patterns of the neurocentral synchondrosis (NCS) in immature cadaveric vertebra. J Pediatr Orthop. 2018;38(3):181–4. https://doi.org/10.1097/BPO.0000000000000781.
5. Abelin-Genevois K, Idjerouidene A, Roussouly P, et al. Cervical spine alignment in the paediatric population a radiographic normative study of 150 asymptomatic patients. Eur Spine J. 2014;23:1442–8.
6. Lustrin ES, Karakas SP, Ortiz AO, et al. Pediatric cervical spine: normal anatomy, variants and trauma. Radiographics. 2003;23:539–60.
7. Cronin CG, Lohan DG, Ni Mhuircheartigh J, et al. MRI evaluation and measurement of the normal odontoid peg position. Clin Radiol. 2007;62:897–903.
8. Baysal B, Eser MB, Sorkun M. Radiological approach to basilar invagination type B: reliability and accuracy. J Neuroradiol. 2020;49:33–49. https://doi.org/10.1016/j.neurad.2020.08.005.
9. Xu S, Gong R. Clivodens angle: a new diagnostic method for basilar invagination at computed tomography. Spine. 2016;41(17):1365–71.
10. Elliott S. The odontoid process in children—is it hypoplastic? Clin Radiol. 1988;39:391–3.
11. Gaunt T, Mankad K, Calder A, Tan AP, Talenti G, Watson TA, Thompson D. Abnormalities of the craniovertebral junction in the paediatric population: a novel biomechanical approach. Clin Radiol. 2018;73:839–54. https://doi.org/10.1016/j.crad.2018.05.020.
12. Locke GR, Gardner JI, Van Epps EF. Atlas-dens interval (ADI) in children. Am J Radiol. 1966;97(1):135.
13. Kale SS, Ailawadhi P, Yerramneni VK, et al. Paediatric bony craniovertebral junction abnormalities: institutional experience of 10 years. J Paediatr Neurosci. 2011;6(Suppl1):S91–5.
14. Keats TE, Sistrom C. Atlas of radiological measurement. 7th ed. Philadelphia, PA: Harcourt Health Services; 2001. p. 141–2.

15. Ghanem I, Hage SE, Rachkidi R, et al. Pediatric cervical spine instability. J Child Orthop. 2008;2:71–84. https://doi.org/10.1007/s11832-008-0092-2.
16. Vermess D, Rojas CA, Shaheen F, Pinakpani R, Martinez CR. Normal pediatric prevertebral soft-tissue thickness on MDCT. Am J Roentgenol. 2012;199:W130–3.
17. Johnson KT, Al-Holou WN, Anderson RCE, et al. Morphometric analysis of the developing pediatric cervical spine. J Neurosurg Pediatr. 2016;18:377–89.
18. Wang JC, Nuccion SL, Feighan JE, et al. Growth and development of the pediatric cervical spine documented radiologically. J Bone Jt Surg. 2001;83(8):1212–8.
19. Kim H, Kim HS, Moon ES, Yoon CS, Chung TS, Song HT, Suh JS, Lee YH, Kim S. Scoliosis imaging: what radiologists should know. Radiographics. 2010;30(7):1823–42. https://doi.org/10.1148/rg.307105061.
20. Roussouly P, Nnadi C. Sagittal plane deformity: an overview of interpretation and management. Eur Spine J. 2010;19(11):1824–36. https://doi.org/10.1007/s00586-010-1476-9. Epub 2010 Jun 22
21. Society of Scoliosis Research. Conditions and treatment. 2022. https://www.srs.org/professionals/online-education-and-resources/conditions-and-treatments.
22. Papp T, Porter RW, Aspden RM. The growth of the lumbar vertebral canal. Spine. 1994;19:2770–3.
23. Watts R. Lumbar vertebral canal size in adults and children: observations from a skeletal sample from London, England. Homo. 2013;64:120–8.
24. Hinck VC, Hopkins CE, Clark WM. Sagittal diameter of the lumbar spinal canal in children and adults. Radiology. 1965;85(5):929–37.
25. Knirsch W, Kurtz C, Häffner N, Langer M, Kececioglu D. Normal values of the sagittal diameter of the lumbar spine (vertebral body and dural sac) in children measured by MRI. Pediatr Radiol. 2005;35(4):419–24. Epub 2005 Jan 6. https://doi.org/10.1007/s00247-004-1382-6.

Shoulder

Chiara Giraudo and Giulia Fichera

Introduction

The shoulder is a very important joint from a structural and functional point of view. It has a complex development which begins during the fourth week of embryonic life [1, 2]. At birth, the humeral diaphysis, the midportion of the clavicle, and the body of the scapula are ossified [1, 2]. Multiple secondary ossification centers appear and ossify at different timepoints with the medial physis of the clavicle usually being the last to reach complete closure by around 20–25 years of age [3]. The regular development of the elements of the joint is essential to guarantee stability and proper function as it is the case of the glenoid version [4]. Thus, a deep knowledge of typical radiological features and measurements of the pediatric shoulder taking into account the physiological changes at different ages is crucial to avoid the potential misinterpretation

C. Giraudo (✉)
Unit of Advanced Clinical and Translational Imaging, Department of Medicine—DIMED, University of Padova, Padova, Italy
e-mail: chiara.giraudo@unipd.it

G. Fichera
Pediatric Radiology Unit, Hospital of Padova, Padova, Italy

P. Simoni, M. P. Aparisi Gómez (eds.), *Essential Measurements in Pediatric Musculoskeletal Imaging*,
https://doi.org/10.1007/978-3-031-17735-4_4

of normal findings [5]. Therefore, the aim of this chapter is to provide a comprehensive overview of the main measurements that can support the radiologist in assessing the various components of this joint in children.

Proximal Humerus and Glenohumeral Joint

Humeral Metaphyseal Stripe

In the metaphysis of long bones of children and young adults, there is a layer of subperiosteal fibrovascular tissue which can be easily detected by magnetic resonance imaging (MRI). This finding has been initially described in the posterior part of the distal femur, but its presence is now well-known also in the humerus. It is characterized by a thin line of 1–2 mm thickness, hyperintense on fluid-sensitive images, and with intermediate signal on T1w imaging (Fig. 1). It runs parallel to the proximal humeral cortex of the metaphyseal region separating it from the periosteum. It can be seen in patients up to around 15 years of age. Less frequently, the humeral metaphyseal stripe can be identified also in the distal clavicle and acromion [5, 6].

Glenoid Version

The anteroposterior glenoid angle, also known as glenoid version, changes during childhood. In fact, in children younger than 2 years, there is usually a slight retroversion or anteversion (approximately ±6°) with a higher prevalence of the former (68% vs. 32%) [1, 7]. The glenoid is most retroverted during the first 2 years of life (-6.3 +/- 6.5 degrees) and by the end of the first decade of life reaches adult glenoid version (-1.7 +/- 6.4 degrees) [7]. The glenoid version plays an important role in the diagnosis of glenoid hypoplasia or dysplasia and glenohumeral instability. Glenoid hypoplasia is due to an incomplete ossification of the inferior ossification center of

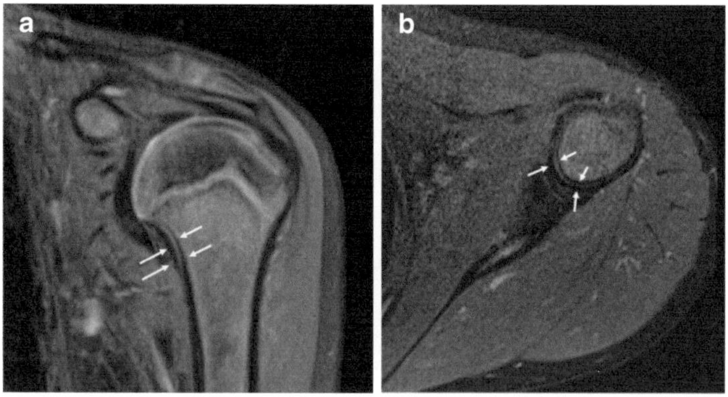

FIGURE 1 Coronal (**a**) and axial (**b**) fat saturated proton density magnetic resonance image of the left shoulder of a 6-year-old boy nicely demonstrating the humeral metaphyseal stripe which is characterized by a thin hyperintense line (normal range 1–2 mm) due to the presence of fibrovascular tissue

the glenoid which can then in turn lead to glenohumeral instability [8]. In the past, glenoid hypoplasia was considered a rare condition but nowadays a prevalence of 18–35% is reported [8]. Glenoid dysplasia can be associated with brachial plexus birth palsy and in these patients, a retroverted glenoid is frequently detected [9]. The glenoid version is commonly assessed by the Friedman method which was first applied in 1992 and is based on three landmarks identified on axial CT images (landmarks can also be identified on MRI) (Fig. 2) [10, 11]. Ditzler and colleagues proposed a modified version using a reference point related to the acromion-scapular body interface which demonstrated to be robust and reproducible [10].

Yellin and colleagues, using MR arthrography, suggested the application of the glenoid index (i.e., glenoid height-to-width ratio), already validated in adults, for children. In their population (55 children <19 years old), they found greater glenoid indexes in patients with anterior glenohumeral dislocation and demonstrated that values ≥1.45 had good specificity (83%) and sensitivity (79%) in predicting joint dislocation [12].

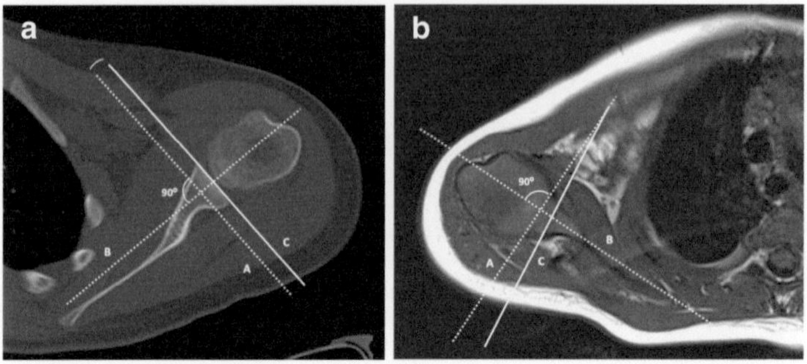

FIGURE 2 (**a**) Axial computed tomography of the left shoulder of a 13-year-old boy with standard anteroposterior glenoid angle measured according to the method of Friedman. The angle is measured between a line perpendicular (*A*) to the main scapular axis (*B*) and a line connecting the anterior and posterior margins of the glenoid (*C*) [10, 11]. (**b**) The Friedman angle demonstrates slight retroversion on the axial T1 magnetic resonance image of the right shoulder of a 20-month-old boy

Acromioclavicular Joint and Coracoclavicular Ligament

The acromioclavicular joint is a small joint of 9 mm height, 19 mm length, and around 1–7 mm width [13, 14]. A widened acromioclavicular joint above 8 mm suggests rupture of the acromioclavicular ligaments (Fig. 3).

Nevertheless, it should be underlined that upper limb injuries in children younger than 13 years rarely cause a complete dislocation of the acromioclavicular joint (<10% of the cases) [15] but rather determine a fracture of the growth plate of the distal clavicle [16]. On the contrary, adolescents usually sustain acromioclavicular dislocation, similarly to adults.

It should not be overlooked that in children, an apparent widening of the acromioclavicular joint can be seen up to the

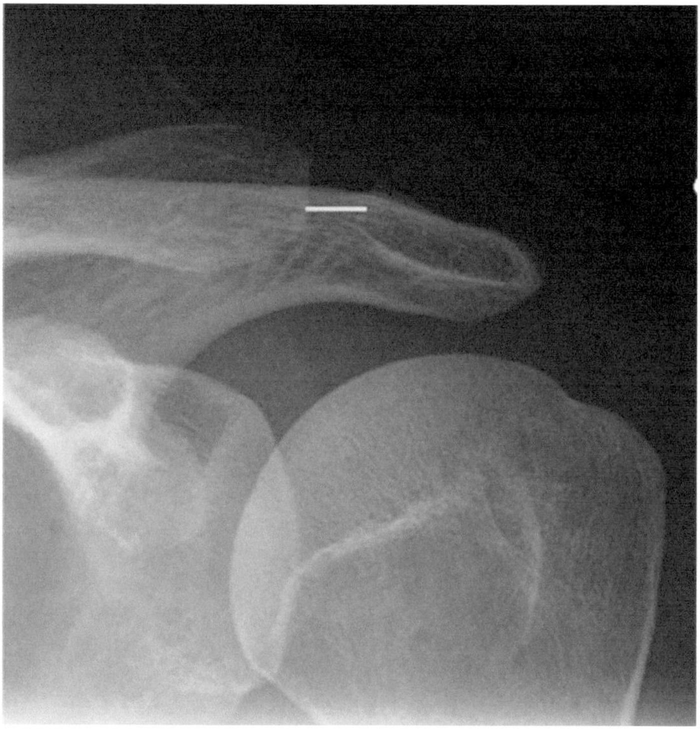

FIGURE 3 Regular acromioclavicular joint distance (<8 mm) measured on the anteroposterior X-ray of the left shoulder of a 13-year-old boy. This type of measurement can be performed also on the Zanca view with a cranial tilting of about 10–15° [3]

time of ossification of the distal acromion and clavicle (i.e., 18–25 years of age) and may mimic an acromioclavicular separation [5] (Fig. 4).

At X-ray, the Zanca view (10°–15° cephalic tilt and lower kV than for the standard AP view), centered on the acromioclavicular joint and without superimposition of the clavicle and the scapula, is recommended to assess this joint [3].

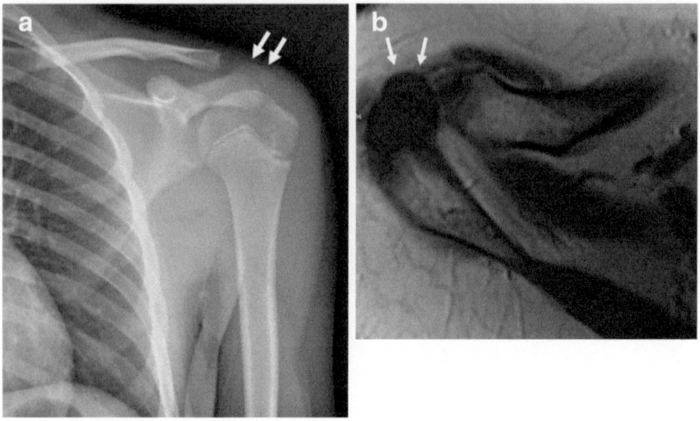

FIGURE 4 (**a**) Anteroposterior X-ray of the shoulder of a 13-year-old boy demonstrating widening of the left acromioclavicular joint due to the still incomplete ossification of the distal clavicle and acromion (white arrows) which should not be misinterpreted as pathological. (**b**) The axial T1-weighted turbo spin echo magnetic resonance image of the right nicely shows the incomplete ossification of the distal acromion in an 11-year-old boy (white arrows)

Regarding the coracoclavicular distance, the normal range is usually between 11 and 13 mm with higher values suggesting a ligament rupture [16, 17] (Fig. 5). The coracoclavicular distance can be assessed on the anteroposterior X-ray view as well as on coronal CT and MR images. Performing comparison views could be useful in differentiating between normal variations and pathological findings [17]. The coracoclavicular ratio, obtained by comparing coracoclavicular distances amongst both sides, can be used to evaluate vertical displacement in patients with suspected acromioclavicular joint separations. On X-ray, an additional method based on the use of the Zanca view and comparative measure-

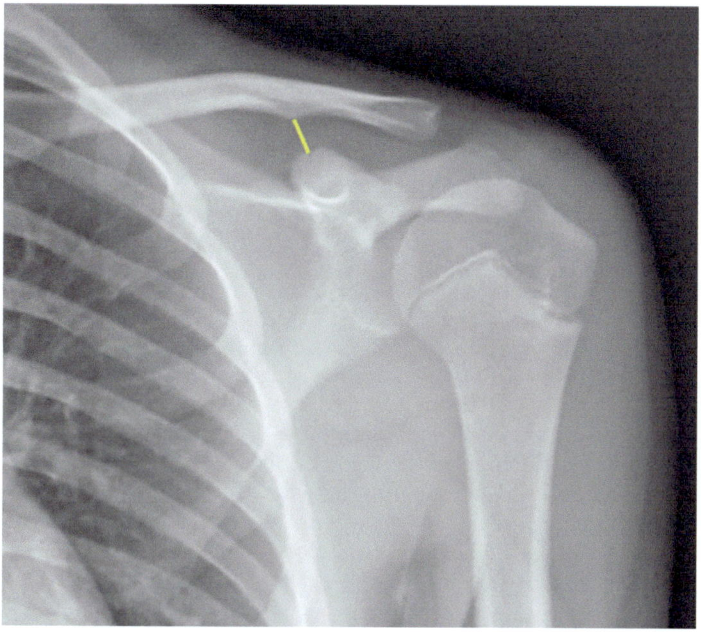

FIGURE 5 Anteroposterior radiograph of the shoulder demonstrating the regular coracoclavicular distance (values >13 mm suggest rupture of the ligament)

ments on both sides may be performed. The D/A ratio (Fig. 6) (*A* being the height of the acromion, between its inferior and superior margins and *D* the distance between a line drawn through the inferior margin of the acromion and a parallel line passing through the lowest and most lateral point of the clavicle) is 0% in normal alignment (*D* should be 0). The value of the ratio (in %) is a measurement of the joint displacement normalised for the "radiological thickness" of the acromion [18].

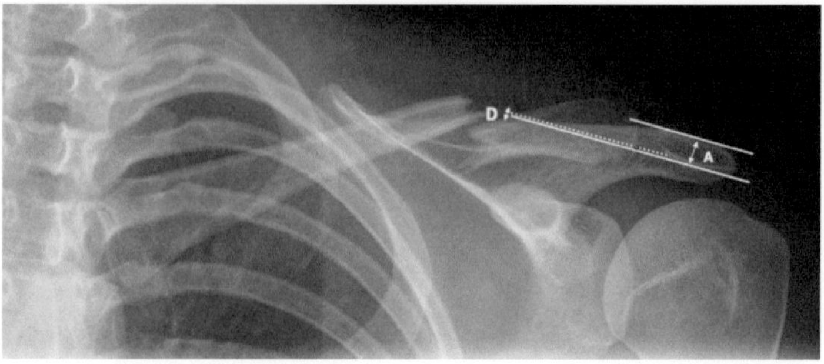

FIGURE 6 Zanca's view in a 15-year-old girl. There is a displaced fracture of the left clavicule. In some cases the coracoclavicular distance may be distorted, not useful to assess acromioclavicular alignment. The *D/A* ratio in this case is 0% (normal). This rules out a luxation of the acromioclavicular joint. *A*, height of the acromion, between its inferior and superior margins. *D*, distance between a line drawn through the inferior margin of the acromion and a parallel line passing through the lowest and most lateral point of the clavicle (dotted yellow line)

References

1. Chauvin NA, Jaimes C, Laor T, Jaramillo D. Magnetic resonance imaging of the pediatric shoulder. Magn Reson Imaging Clin N Am. 2012;20(2):327–47.
2. Rockwood CA. The shoulder. 4th ed. Philadelphia: Saunders/Elsevier; 2009.
3. Flores DV, Goes PK, Gomez CM, Umpire DF, Pathria MN. Imaging of the acromioclavicular joint: anatomy, function, pathologic features, and treatment. Radiographics. 2020;40(5):1355–82.
4. Palmer W, Bancroft L, Bonar F, Choi JA, Cotten A, Griffith JF, et al. Glossary of terms for musculoskeletal radiology. Skeletal Radiol. 2020;49(Suppl 1):S1–S33.
5. Zember J, Rosenberg ZS, Kwong S, Kothary SP, Bedoya MA. Normal skeletal maturation and imaging pitfalls in the pediatric shoulder. Radiographics. 2015;35(4):1108–22.

6. Kwong S, Kothary S, Poncinelli LL. Skeletal development of the proximal Humerus in the pediatric population: MRI features. Am J Roentgenol. 2014;202(2):418–25.
7. Mintzer CM, Waters PM, Brown DJ. Glenoid version in children. J Pediatr Orthop. 1996;16(5):563–6.
8. Baca MJ, King RW, Bancroft LW. Glenoid hypoplasia. Radiol Case Rep. 2016;11(4):386–90.
9. Chagas-Neto FA, Dalto VF, Crema MD, Waters PM, Gregio-Junior E, Mazzer N, et al. Imaging assessment of glenohumeral dysplasia secondary to brachial plexus birth palsy. Radiol Bras. 2016;49(3):144–9.
10. Ditzler MG, Herman Kan J, Artunduaga M, Jadhav SP, Bell BR, Zhang W, et al. Modified Friedman technique: a new proposed method of measuring glenoid version in the setting of glenohumeral dysplasia. Pediatr Radiol. 2018;48(12):1779–85.
11. Amadi HO, Banerejee S, Hansen UN, Wallace AN, Bull AMJ. An optimised method for quantifying glenoid orientation. Int J Shoulder Surg. 2008;2(2):25–9.
12. Yellin JL, Fabricant PD, Anari JB, Neuwirth AL, Ganley T, Chauvin NA, et al. Increased glenoid index as a risk factor for pediatric and adolescent anterior Glenohumeral dislocation. Orthop J Sports Med. 2021;9(3):2325967120986139.
13. Frank RM, Cotter EJ, Leroux TS, Romeo AA. Acromioclavicular joint injuries: evidence-based treatment. J Am Acad Orthop Surg. 2019;27(17):e775–88.
14. Petersson CJ, Redlund-Johnell I. Radiographic joint space in normal acromioclavicular joints. Acta Orthop Scand. 1983;54(3):431–3.
15. Karantanas AH, Baert AL. Sports injuries in children and adolescents. 1st ed. Cham: Springer Nature; 2011.
16. Eidman DK, Siff SJ, Tullos HS. Acromioclavicular lesions in children. Am J Sports Med. 1981;9(3):150–4.
17. Alyas F, Curtis M, Speed C, Saifuddin A, Connell D. MR imaging appearances of acromioclavicular joint dislocation. Radiographics. 2008;28(2):463–79.
18. Gastaud O, Raynier JL, Duparc F, Baverel L, Andrieu K, Tarissi N, et al. Reliability of radiographic measurements for acromioclavicular joint separations. Orthop Traumatol Surg Res. 2015;101(8 Suppl):S291–5.

Elbow

Riccardo De Angelis and Paolo Simoni

Introduction

Technique and Quality Assessment

Anteroposterior (AP) and lateral (LAT) radiographs of the elbow should be always performed. Additional oblique views should be performed, when necessary. Accurate placement is essential to avoid inaccurate measurements.

In the anteroposterior view, the elbow is extended, and the forearm is fully supinated.

A true lateral projection is required in lateral view, with the elbow flexed by 90°, the forearm in a neutral position, and the arm perpendicular to the coronal plane of the patient, with the thumb directed upward [1]. Good anteroposterior

R. De Angelis
Diagnostic Imaging, Institut Bordet, Brussels, Belgium

Pediatric Imaging Department, Reine Fabiola Children's University Hospital, Université libre de Bruxelles, Brussels, Belgium

P. Simoni (✉)
Pediatric Imaging Department, Reine Fabiola Children's University Hospital, Université libre de Bruxelles, Brussels, Belgium

P. Simoni, M. P. Aparisi Gómez (eds.), *Essential Measurements in Pediatric Musculoskeletal Imaging*,
https://doi.org/10.1007/978-3-031-17735-4_5

radiographs should always show a true frontal view of distal humerus (Fig. 1, number *1*), the humero-radial joint space, and epiphyseal cartilage (Fig. 1, number *2*).

To assess the radiograph quality on the lateral view, the AABCS the systematic approach based can be used [2]:

- A: *Adequacy*—Check the presence of an "hourglass" appearance of the distal humerus. If the "hourglass" is not symmetrical, the view is rotated.
- A: *Alignment*—The anterior humeral line (see below) paralleling the anterior cortex of the humerus must cross the middle third of the capitellum. The radiocapitellar line (see below), parallels the radial neck on the AP and lateral views and should always cross the capitellum.
- B: *Bone*—Examine each bone for cortical abnormalities. Check the number and the position of the ossification centers.

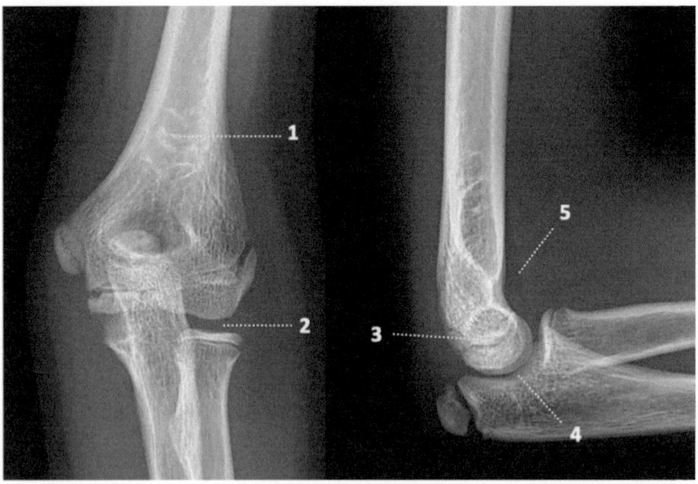

Figure 1 Assessement of radiograph quality: radiographs should always show a frontal view of distal humerus (*1*) and humero-radial joint space (*2*) on anteroposterior view, as well as perfect condylar superposition on lateral view (*3*), a view of the articular space (*4*) and fat pad (*5*)

- C: *Cartilage*—Inspect the joint space to determine whether they are enlarged. Consider the presence of the epiphyseal radiolucent cartilage in children.
- S: *Soft tissue*—The anterior fat pad is usually concealed within the coronoid fossa, but sometimes may be seen, parallel to the anterior humeral line. This can be lifted due to the presence of effusion (anterior fat pad sign or sail sign). Visualization of a posterior fat pad indicates the existence of an effusion (lifting the fat pad, posterior fat pad sign), given this is normally not seen on the true lateral projection.

A good lateral view should always present a perfect condylar superposition (Fig. 1, number *3*), a view of articular space (Fig. 1, number *4*), and a view of the anterior fat pad (Fig. 1, number *5*).

Ossification Centers

Six ossification centers are located around the elbow. It is essential to know the exact order of appearance since it will help on detecting fractures and other irregularities, using the mnemonic CRITOE. This systematic approach is mandatory to avoid overcalling fractures in children (see Table 1 and Fig. 2) [3].

To remember the age of appearance of the ossification centers, two numerical successions can be used [4]:

A simple numerical successions to remember for the CRITOE is 1, 3, 5, 7, 9, and 11 years of age (see Table 1).

In adolescents, these ossification centers fuse.

The mnemonic "CTE-R-O-I" can be of help to remember the order in which they fuse [4]:

- CTE: At the age of 13, the capitulum, trochlea, and external (lateral) epicondyle become a unique center.
- R-O-I: The radius, olecranon, and internal (medial) epicondyle integrate with the CTE at the ages of 15, 16, and 17, respectively.

Table 1 Order and average age of appearance of elbow ossification centers

CRITOE mnemonic						
	C	**R**	**I**	**T**	**O**	**E**
Ossification center	Capitellum	Radius	Internal epicondyle	Trochlea	Olecranon	External epicondyle
Age of appearance	1–3 years	3–5 years	3–5 years	5–7 years	7–9 years	9–11 years

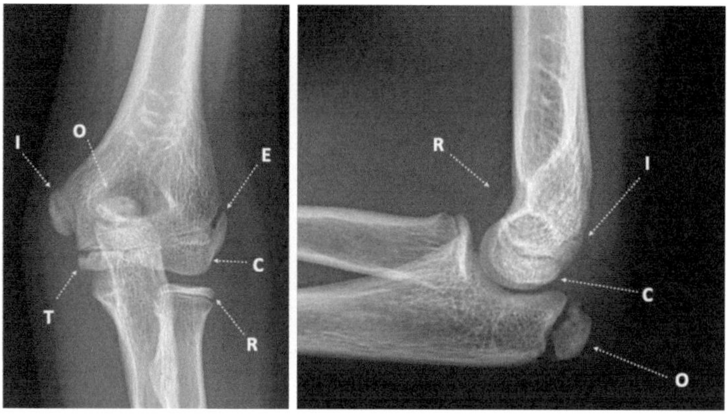

FIGURE 2 The mnemonic CRITOE can help remember the exact order of appearance of elbow ossification centers

The Anterior Humeral Line (AHL)

- In the lateral view, the AHL is drawn along the anterior cortex of the humerus (Fig. 3a). It crosses the middle third of the humeral condyle.
- In children over the age of 5, the AHL crosses the middle third of the capitellum. However, there is considerable variation in children under the age of 5: In 25% of those children, the AHL passes through the anterior third of the humeral condyle. A posterior displacement of the capitellum relative to the AHL can suggest a fracture.
- AHL as a reference may not be sufficient to detect an elbow fracture because this line does not reach the central third of the capitellum in up to 49% of normal elbows, with variation depending on patient age [5]. Noticeably, in up to 30% of children before 2 years of age, the AHL passes through the anterior third of the humeral capitellum ossification center [6].

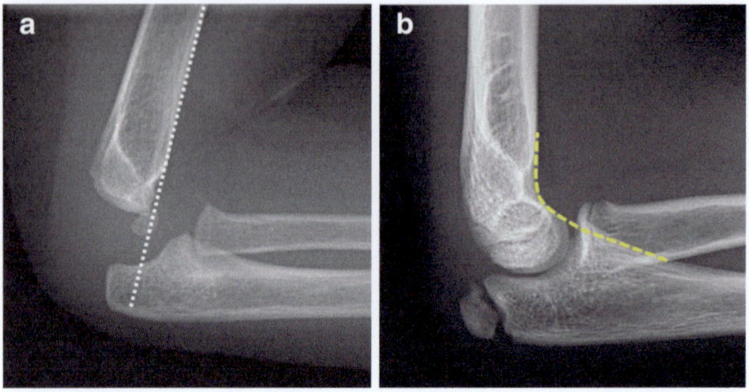

FIGURE 3 The anterior humeral line (**a**) and the anterior coronoid line (**b**)

The Anterior Coronoid Line

- The anterior coronoid line (ACL) is a curved line visible on the lateral view. The ACL follows the anterior aspect of the ulna, over the coronoid, to the anterior aspect of the distal humeral shaft (Fig. 3b).
- ACL can be used to assess articular congruency in a glace [7].

Shaft Condylar Angle (SCA)

- The shaft condylar angle (SCA) might be used to complement the AHL measurement. The SCA is defined as the angle formed between the axis of the distal humerus shaft and the line bisecting the humeral condyle (Fig. 4a).
- The normal value for SCA is of 40.10° ± 6.24° [8].
- An abnormal SCA is indicative of a supracondylar fracture [9].

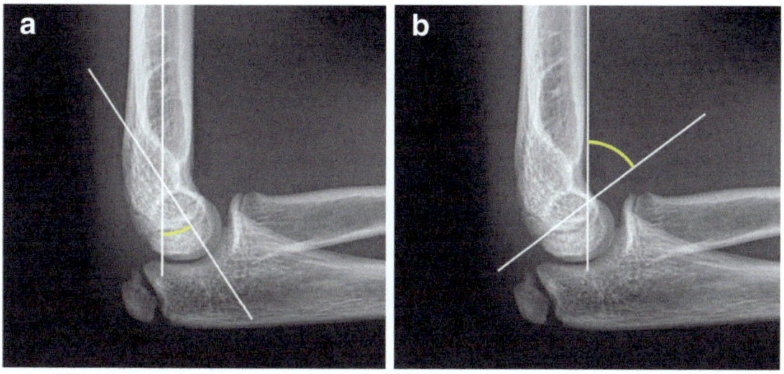

FIGURE 4 Shaft condylar angle (**a**) and lateral capitellohumeral angle (**b**)

Lateral Capitellohumeral Angle (LCHA)

The lateral capitellohumeral angle (LCHA) is formed by a line drawn along the anterior aspect of the humerus and a line passing along the growth plate of the capitellum (Fig. 4b) [8].

The value reported for LCHA for children is 47.79° ± 5.13°.

The Radiocapitellar Line

- The radiocapitellar line (RCL) is the midline of the proximal radius. On normal radiographs, it should cross the ossification center of the capitellum (Fig. 5).
- The RCL does not cross the capitellum ossification center in case of luxation [10].

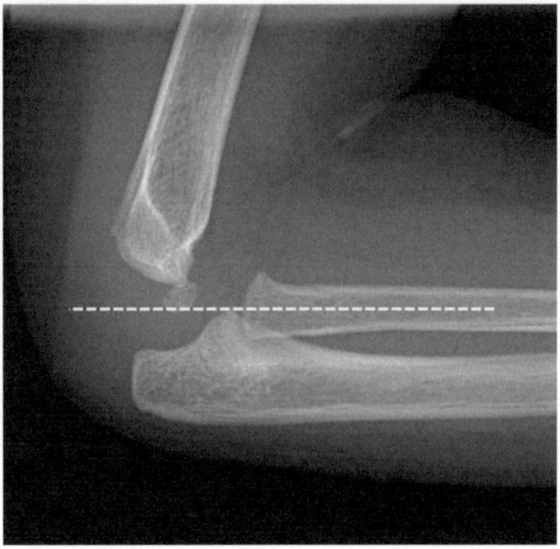

FIGURE 5 Radiocapitellar line

Humeral and Ulnar Shaft Lines

Measured in the AP view, the humeral and ulnar shaft lines are along the longitudinal axis of the humeral and ulnar shafts, respectively (Fig. 6). In fractures or other deformations, the normal spatial relations between the humeral and ulnar shaft lines are frequently lost.

The Carrying Angle

- On AP view, this is the angle formed by the humeral shaft line and the ulnar shaft line (Fig. 6a).
- In males, the normal values are 11–14°, whereas in females, values are 13–16° [11].
- In case of a reduced carrying angle, the forearm may point medially. This is also known as Gunstock deformity, or cubitus varus, and is a frequent complication of supracondylar fractures [12].

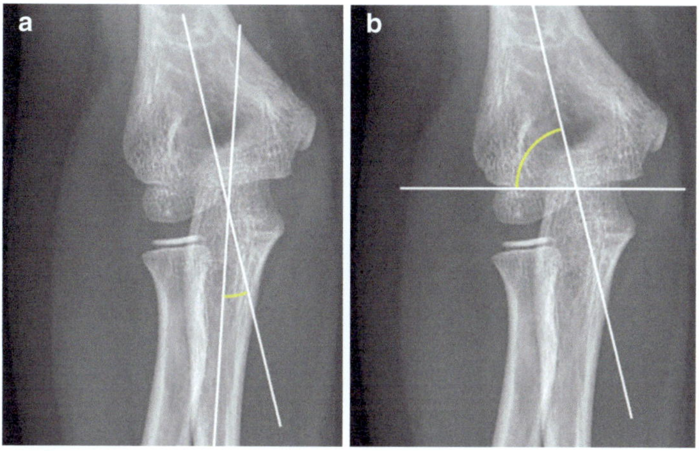

FIGURE 6 Carrying angle (**a**) and Baumann's angle (**b**)

Baumann's Angle

- Baumann's angle, also known as the humeral-capitellar angle, is measured on the AP view.
- Baumann's angle is defined by the intersection of a line drawn along the growth plate of the capitellum and a line drawn along the long axis of the humeral shaft (Fig. 6b).
- The normal range of Baumann's angle is 70–75° [13].
- In adolescents, as the lateral condyle begins to fuse with the distal humerus, Baumann's angle may be difficult to measure. Therefore, in case of doubt, it should be compared to the opposite elbow [14].
- Baumann's angle is used to determine displacement in supracondylar humeral fractures [15].

Medial Epicondyle-Epiphyseal (MEE) Angle

- The medial epicondyle-epiphyseal angle (MEE) is formed by the intersection of a line drawn along the long axis of the humeral shaft and a line passing along the medial epicondylar growth plate (Fig. 7).

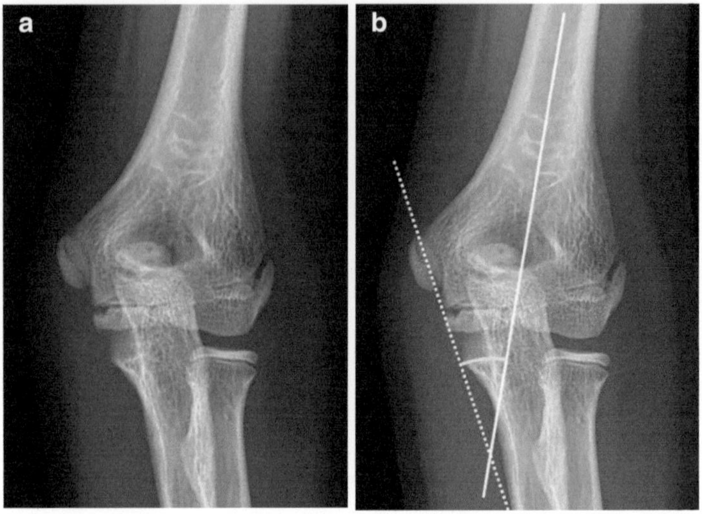

FIGURE 7 Medial epicondyle-epiphyseal (MEE) angle. (**a**) AP view, (**b**) measurement of the angle

- The MEE angle average value is 38.2° ± 4.17°.
- The MEE angle can be used to assess supracondylar fracture reduction on the AP view [16].

References

1. Iyer RS, Thapa MM, Khanna PC, Chew FS. Pediatric bone imaging: imaging elbow trauma in children—a review of acute and chronic injuries. AJR Am J Roentgenol. 2012;198(5):1053–68. PMID: 22528894. https://doi.org/10.2214/AJR.10.7314.
2. DeFroda SF, Hansen H, Gil JA, Hawari AH, Cruz AI Jr. Radiographic evaluation of common pediatric elbow injuries. Orthop Rev. 2017;9(1):7030. PMID: 28286625; PMCID: PMC5337779. https://doi.org/10.4081/or.2017.7030.
3. Underschultz JG, Stagg A, MacGougan CK. Applying CRITOE in pediatric elbow trauma: is that a fracture or an ossification center? CJEM. 2021;23(3):398–400. Epub 2021 Feb 15. PMID: 33587249. https://doi.org/10.1007/s43678-020-00072-w.

4. Patel B, Reed M, Patel S. Gender-specific pattern differences of the ossification centers in the pediatric elbow. Pediatr Radiol. 2009;39(3):226–31. Epub 2009 Jan 6. PMID: 19125245. https://doi.org/10.1007/s00247-008-1078-4.
5. Herman MJ, Boardman MJ, Hoover JR, Chafetz RS. Relationship of the anterior humeral line to the capitellar ossific nucleus: variability with age. J Bone Joint Surg Am. 2009;91(9):2188–93. PMID: 19723996. https://doi.org/10.2106/JBJS.H.01316.
6. Ryan DD, Lightdale-Miric NR, Joiner ER, Wren TA, Spragg L, Heffernan MJ, Kay RM, Skaggs DL. Variability of the anterior humeral line in Normal pediatric elbows. J Pediatr Orthop. 2016;36(2):e14–6. PMID: 26035494. https://doi.org/10.1097/BPO.0000000000000529.
7. Vashisht S, Banerjee S. Cubitus varus. In: Stat pearls. Treasure Island, FL: StatPearls; 2021. PMID: 32809529.
8. Musikachart P, Ariyawatkul T, Wongcharoenwatana J, Piamthipmanas T, Chanchoo S, Eamsobhana P. Intra-observer and inter-observer reliability of shaft condylar angle and lateral Capitellohumeral angle: evaluation based on reliability in different ages and levels of experience. Orthop Surg. 2019;11(3):467–73. PMID: 31243918; PMCID: PMC6595104
9. Sukvanich P, Samun P, Kongmalai P. Diagnostic accuracy of the shaft-condylar angle for an incomplete supracondylar fracture of elbow in children. Eur J Orthop Surg Traumatol. 2019;29(8):1673–7. Epub 2019 Jul 4. PMID: 31273492. https://doi.org/10.1007/s00590-019-02489-1.
10. Sandman E, Canet F, Petit Y, Laflamme GY, Athwal GS, Rouleau DM. Effect of elbow position on radiographic measurements of radio-capitellar alignment. World J Orthop. 2016;7(2):117–22. PMID: 26925383; PMCID: PMC4757656. https://doi.org/10.5312/wjo.v7.i2.117.
11. Balasubramanian P, Madhuri V, Muliyil J. Carrying angle in children: a normative study. J Pediatr Orthop B. 2006;15(1):37–40. PMID: 16280718. https://doi.org/10.1097/01202412-200601000-00008.
12. Golden DW, Jhee JT, Gilpin SP, Sawyer JR. Elbow range of motion and clinical carrying angle in a healthy pediatric population. J Pediatr Orthop B. 2007;16(2):144–9. PMID: 17273043. https://doi.org/10.1097/BPB.0b013e328010fcf2.
13. Keenan WN, Clegg J. Variation of Baumann's angle with age, sex, and side: implications for its use in radiological monitoring of supracondylar fracture of the humerus in children. J Pediatr Orthop. 1996;16(1):97–8. PMID: 8747363. https://doi.org/10.1097/01241398-199601000-00019.

14. Acton JD, McNally MA. Baumann's confusing legacy. Injury. 2001;32(1):41–3. PMID: 11164401. https://doi.org/10.1016/s0020-1383(00)00102-9.
15. Suangyanon P, Chalayon O, Worawuthangkul K, Kaewpornsawan K, Ariyawatkul T, Eamsobhana P. Pediatric elbow measurement parameters: Evaluation of the six angles in inter- and intra-observer reliability. J Clin Orthop Trauma. 2019;10(4):792–6. Epub 2018 Jul 23. PMID: 31316257; PMCID: PMC6612040. https://doi.org/10.1016/j.jcot.2018.07.019.
16. Biyani A, Gupta SP, Sharma JC. Determination of medial epicondylar epiphyseal angle for supracondylar humeral fractures in children. J Pediatr Orthop. 1993;13(1):94–7. PMID: 8416364. https://doi.org/10.1097/01241398-199301000-00019.

Wrist

Gwendolyn Vuurberg, Floor J. M. de Jaeger, Sjoerd Jens, and Mario Maas

G. Vuurberg
Division of Musculoskeletal Radiology, Department of Radiology and Nuclear Medicine, Amsterdam UMC, University of Amsterdam, Amsterdam Movement Sciences, Amsterdam, The Netherlands

Academic Center of Evidence Based Sports Medicine (ACES), Amsterdam, The Netherlands

Department of Radiology and Nuclear Medicine, Rijnstate Hospital, Arnhem, The Netherlands

F. J. M. de Jaeger
Division of Musculoskeletal Radiology, Department of Radiology and Nuclear Medicine, Amsterdam UMC, University of Amsterdam, Amsterdam Movement Sciences, Amsterdam, The Netherlands

S. Jens
Department of Radiology and Nuclear Medicine, Rijnstate Hospital, Arnhem, The Netherlands

P. Simoni, M. P. Aparisi Gómez (eds.), *Essential Measurements in Pediatric Musculoskeletal Imaging*,
https://doi.org/10.1007/978-3-031-17735-4_6

M. Maas (✉)
Division of Musculoskeletal Radiology, Department of Radiology and Nuclear Medicine, Amsterdam UMC, University of Amsterdam, Amsterdam Movement Sciences, Amsterdam, The Netherlands

Academic Center of Evidence Based Sports Medicine (ACES), Amsterdam, The Netherlands
e-mail: m.maas@amsterdamumc.nl

Introduction

Children are prone to wrist injuries due to the increasing complex biomechanical demands during outdoor playing, games, and a variety of sport activities [1, 2]. The high demands required for adult livelihood/work underline the importance of adequate diagnostics after a wrist injury at a young age. A clear understanding of the normal growth of the pediatric wrist and corresponding reference values is essential to assess physiological bone growth and to identify pathology or abnormality in children. It is known that multiple pathologies can impair the growth and development of the radius, ulna, and carpal bones.

The wrist is a complex joint with many osseous and ligamentous structures. It is even more complex in children due to not fully ossified structures which may complicate adequate assessment through conventional imaging methods [3]. Development of the wrist starts during the embryonic period and is completed during adolescence. It starts with the primary ossification in the center of long bones and is completed with the process of secondary ossification that focuses on ossification in the epiphysis and metaphysis. The physis, as the transition zone between the metaphysis and epiphysis, is the weakest area of the growing skeleton and therefore more prone to injury [4]. Due to the changing and growing pediatric skeleton, adult measurement standards are not always applicable to the pediatric population and a different set of reference values is used [5].

Standard radiographic evaluation of the wrist in children includes posterior-anterior (PA) and lateral radiographs. The PA projection is performed with the shoulder in 90° abduction, the elbow is flexed to 90°, and the palm of the hand is placed flat on the X-ray plate with the forearm in neutral position. On an adequate PA radiograph, the third metacarpal is in line with the radial shaft. For the lateral projection, the elbow is abducted to the side, and in 90° flexion. For both views, the shoulder, elbow, and wrist are in the same plane.

Wrist imaging can give additional insight on bone development, age, and growth. This chapter elucidates some of the regularly used radiographic measurements of the pediatric wrist and additionally highlights the reference values.

Scapholunate and Capitolunate Angle Measurements

- Carpal angle measurements are performed on a lateral radiograph and include the scapholunate and capitolunate angles. See Tables 1 and 2 for the age-corrected normal values.

  - Scapholunate angle is the angle between:

    The scaphoid axis (long axis of the scaphoid, *A*).
    The lunate axis (line perpendicular to palmar and dorsal poles, *B*) (see Fig. 1a, b).

TABLE 1 Reference values of scapholunate angle in degrees (mean, range) [5]

Age	Male	Female
6	60.7 (0–82)	63.4 (0–82)
7	70.5 (67–74)	63.3 (37–76)
8	64.3 (51–75)	60 (38–81)
9	60.2 (50–72)	73.7 (72–77)
10	67 (50–76)	70 (63–69)
11	62.5 (57–67)	63 (55–69)
12	58.8 (49–63)	51.6 (34–62)
13	45.2 (33–53)	46 (43–59)
14	46.6 (34–58)	46 (42–49)
15	37.5 (36–39)	47 (46–49)
16	39 (35–42)	42.5 (33–35)

TABLE 2 Reference values of capitolunate angle measured in degrees (mean, range) [5]

Age	Male	Female
4	42 (0–59)	36.9 (0–60)
5	52.9 (49–59)	57 (55–60)
6	56 (51–59)	55.4 (49–62)
7	50.5 (50–51)	47.7 (42–51)
8	41.4 (30–49)	44.5 (38–49)
9	44.2 (31–49)	43 (42–45)
10	37.3 (32–40)	40.5 (39–41)
11	33 (23–37)	22.9 (4–38)
12	33.4 (18–63)	33.2 (18–39)
13	12 (8–18)	10 (1–18)
14	11.9 (4–18)	12.6 (6–18)
15	7.4 (4–18)	7.1 (4–24)
16	18.5 (0–25)	16.5 (0–24)

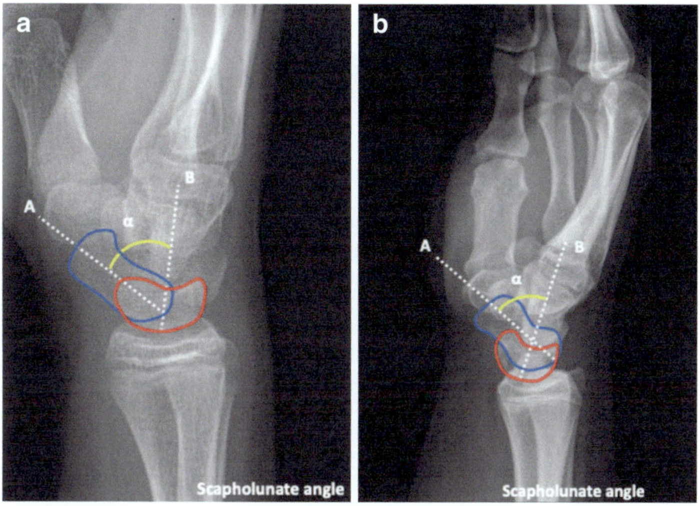

Figure 1 Scapholunate angle. (**a**) 10 years old (**b**) 15 years old

– Capitolunate angle is the angle between:

  The capitate axis (line through central of the proximal and distal articulate surface, *B*).
  The lunate axis (*C*) (Fig. 2a, b).

- Both angles decrease with age until carpal bones are fully ossified. When fully ossified, adult standards can be used [6]. Adult normal values for the scapholunate angle range from 30 to 60 °and for capitolunate angle range from 0 to 30 ° [7].
- Increased scapholunate angle and capitolunate angle can be seen in carpal instability, mostly due to ligamentous injuries of the wrist [8].

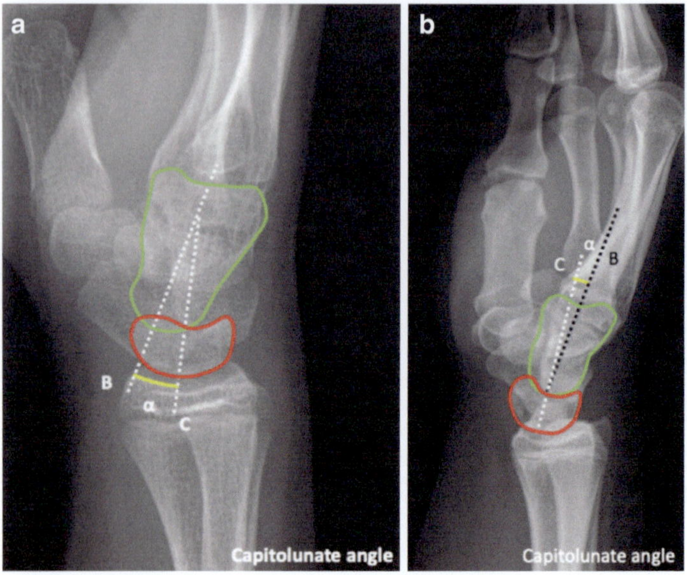

FIGURE 2 Capitolunate angle. (**a**) 10 years old (**b**) 15 years old

Ulnar Variance

- The ulnar variance measurement is used to evaluate the results of fracture treatment. This measurement is performed on a standard PA radiograph of the wrist [9]. See Table 3 for the normal values.
- The ulnar variance measurement for children is defined as the height difference between the metaphyses (Hafner method) or between the articular surfaces (perpendicular method) of the distal radius and distal ulna:
  - The Hafner method can be applied in two ways.

TABLE 3 Age standards of ulnar variance in millimeters (mean, range) measured through the Hafner method and perpendicular method [5, 10]

	Hafner method (mean, range)		Perpendicular method (mean, range)	
Age	Measurement PRPR	Measurement DIDI	Male	Female
2	2.1 (0.3 to 3.8)	2.3 (0.7 to 4.1)		
3	2.1 (0 to 4.2)	2.4 (0.3 to 4.5)		
4	2.1 (−0.3 to 4.6)	2.4 (0 to 4.8)		
5	2.1 (−0.6 to 4.9)	2.4 (−0.2 to 5.2)		
6	2.1 (−0.9 to 5.1)	2.5 (−0.4 to 5.2)		
7	2.2 (−1.1 to 5.4)	2.5 (−0.6 to 5.7)		
8	2.2 (−1.3 to 5.6)	2.5 (−0.8 to 6.0)		
9	2.2 (−1.4 to 5.9)	2.6 (−1.0 to 6.2)		
10	2.2 (−1.6 to 6.1)	2.6 (−1.1 to 6.5)	−2.4 (−2.9 to 1.7)	−2.8 (−4.6 to −1.7)
11	2.2 (−1.8 to 6.3)	2.6 (−1.3 to 6.7)	−2.5 (−3.6 to −1.4)	−2 (−3 to −1)
12	2.2 (−2.0 to 6.5)	2.7 (−1.4 to 6.9)	−2.5 (−4.7 to 0)	−3 (−5 to −1)
13	2.2 (−2.2 to 6.7)	2.7 (−1.5 to 7.1)	−2.4 (−4.9 to 0)	−2.8 (−4 to 0)
14	2.3 (−2.4 to 7.0)	2.7 (−1.7 to 7.3)	−3.1 (−5 to 2.8)	−3.9 (−4.5 to −3)
15	2.3 (−2.4 to 7.0)	2.8 (−1.8 to 7.5)	0.3 (−2.3 to 2.8)	0.3 (−6.1 to 2.8)
16			0 (−1 to 1.2)	0 (−1.5 to 1.6)

Proximal measurement (PRPR): distance between ulnar metaphysis on the radial side (*A*) and radial metaphysis on the ulnar side (*B*) (Fig. 3a, b).
Distal measurement (DIDI): distance between the most distal point of the ulnar metaphysis (*A*) and the most distal point of the radial metaphysis (*B*) [10] (Fig. 4a, b).

– Perpendicular method: distance from the articular surface of the radius (*A*) on the ulnar side to the distal ulnar articular surface (*B*). These lines are drawn perpendicular to the line through the longitudinal axis of the radius [11, 12] (Fig. 5a, b).

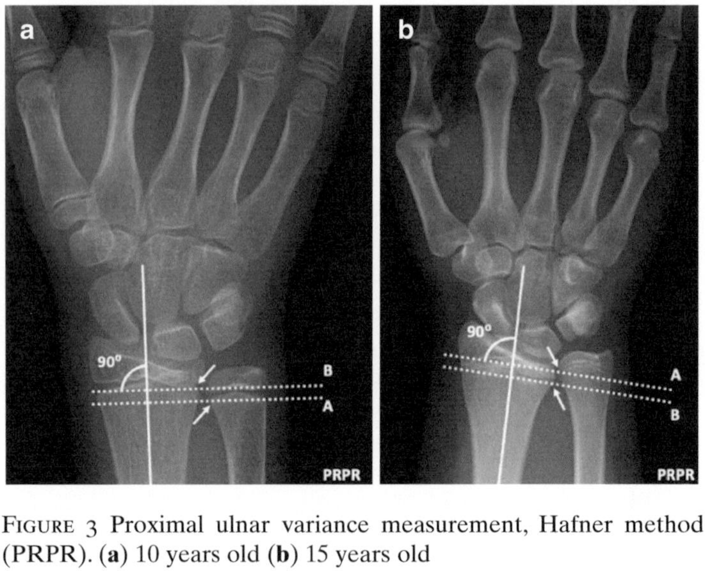

FIGURE 3 Proximal ulnar variance measurement, Hafner method (PRPR). (**a**) 10 years old (**b**) 15 years old

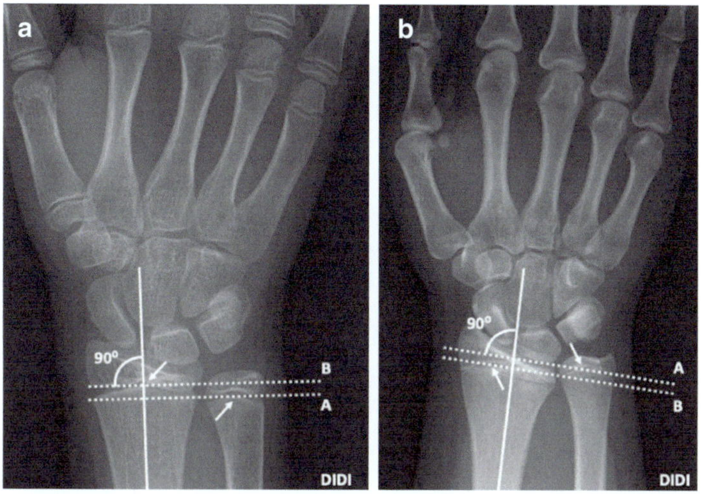

FIGURE 4 Distal ulnar variance measurement, Hafner method (DIDI). (**a**) 10 years old (**b**) 15 years old

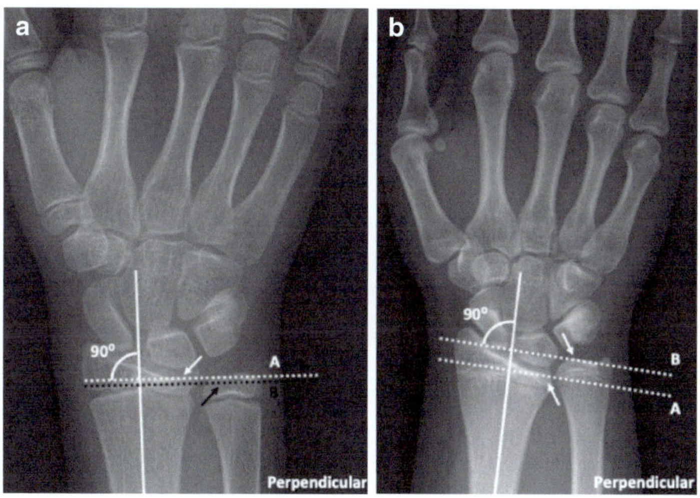

FIGURE 5 Perpendicular method of ulnar variance measurement. (**a**) 10 years old (**b**) 15 years old

  - Kox et al. [13] found that ulnar variance should be measured through the Hafner method in children with open growth plates and a skeletal age of 13 years. The adapted perpendicular method is recommended for a skeletal age of 14 years or older.

- Outcome ulnar variance.
  - Positive = ulna is longer compared to the radius.
  - Neutral = both surfaces are in line.
  - Negative = the ulna is shorter compared to the radius.
- Interpretation of outcome.
  - Positive ulnar variance is associated with ulnar impaction syndrome and degeneration of the triangular fibrocartilage complex (TFCC) following tears [14, 15].
  - Negative ulnar variance may be associated with Kienböck's disease (avascular necrosis of lunate bone) and ulnar impingement syndrome [16–18].
- Ulnar variance (positive and negative) can be the result of trauma, be congenital or be dependent of joint position (both maximum pronation and/or firm grip increase ulnar variance) [16].
- Ulnar variance is otherwise known as Hulten variance or radioulnar index.

Radial Height

- The radial height is measured on a standard PA radiograph of the wrist with the forearm in neutral position. See Table 4 for the age standard.

TABLE 4 Age standards of radial height measured in millimeters (mean, range) [5]

Age	Male	Female
1	7.1 (0–9.8)	5 (0–9.5)
2	8.6 (6.5–9.6)	8.4 (7.6–8.3)
3	7.6 (7.1–8.1)	8.2 (7.6–8.7)
4	8.9 (6.2–11.4)	8 (6.1–8.5)
5	8.4 (4.5–9.6)	8.4 (5.2–9.6)
6	8 (4–10.2)	8.8 (4.8–9.8)
7	9.4 (9.3–10.5)	9 (8.2–9.5)
8	10 (7.8–12.7)	12.5 (8.5–14.4)
9	10.5 (7.6–12.9)	9.7 (7.8–10.7)
10	10.9 (10.4–11.7)	9 (8.4–11.6)
11	11.9 (10–14)	12.3 (10–15)
12	13.5 (11–15)	13.2 (10.7–14.9)
13	13.1 (10–15.8)	12.7 (9–15)
14	11.4 (9.8–14)	10.3 (8–12)
15	10 (6.6–11.4)	9 (6.6–11.4)
16	13.4 (12.2–14.2)	12.3 (8.5–14.2)

- Radial height measurement is measured perpendicular to the radial axis and is in children defined as the distance between:
  - The metaphyseal line, i.e., the most distal point of the radial metaphysis (*A*).
  - The distal tip of the styloid. When the radial styloid has not yet been ossified, the most distal point of the radial epiphysis is used (*C*) [5] (Fig. 6a, b).
- Radial height measurements in children differ from adult measurements because the distal physis complicates the radial height measurement [19].

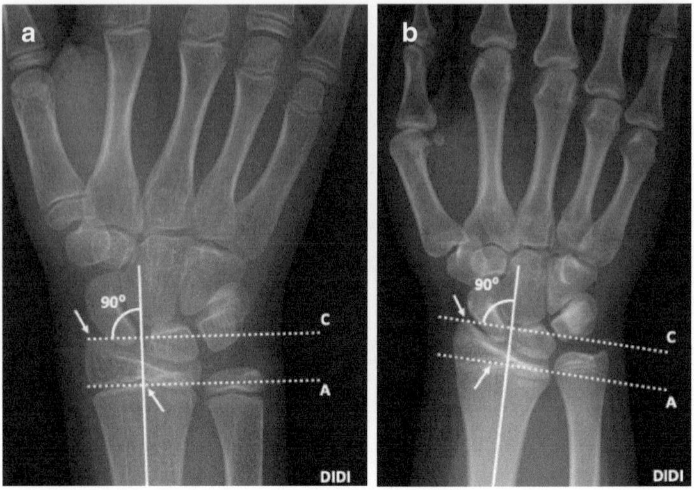

FIGURE 6 Radial height measurement. (**a**) 10 years old. (**b**) 15 years old

- Loss of radial height following a distal radius fracture is associated with poor function of the wrist, mainly due to pain and instability [20, 21].
- Radial height is also known as radial length.

Radial Inclination

- Radial inclination is measured on a standard PA radiograph of the wrist with the forearm in neutral position. See Table 5 for the age standards.
- Radial inclination is defined as the angle between:
  - The line from the radial styloid tip to the ulnar aspect of the distal radius (*D*).
  - The line perpendicular to the long axis of the radius (*A*) [5, 22] (Fig. 7a, b).

TABLE 5 Age standards of radial inclination measured in degrees (mean, range) [5]

Age	Male	Female
4	9.6 (0–17)	7.8 (0–16)
5	11.1 (0–22)	10.1 (0–18)
6	13.8 (0–22)	13.6 (0–23)
7	14.6 (8–24)	16 (11–23)
8	15.5 (11–27)	14.8 (11–19)
9	16 (9–22)	13.7 (8–22)
10	18.5 (0–32)	21.5 (8–31)
11	23 (11–27)	21.8 (0–34)
12	21.6 (18–31)	21.9 (18–28)
13	24.6 (21–33)	24.3 (21–26)
14	24.9 (21–31)	24 (21–26)
15	19 (10–33)	19.4 (14–26)
16	29.7 (18–31)	26.4 (18–29)

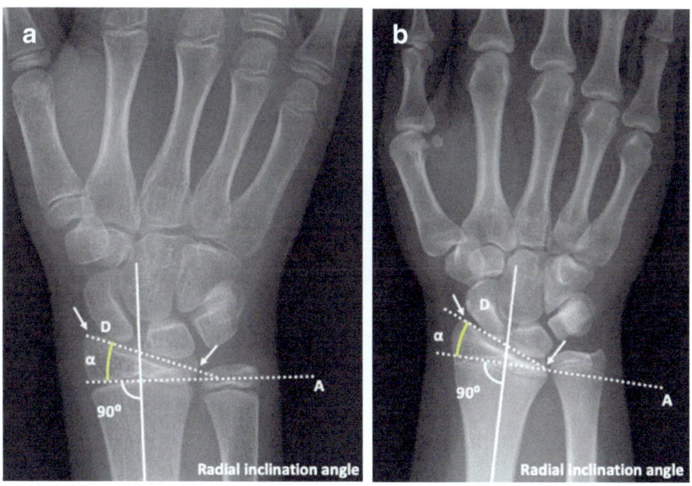

FIGURE 7 Radial inclination measurement. (**a**) 10 years old (**b**) 15 years old

- Loss of radial inclination is associated with loss of radial height and is often a result of a Colles fracture and/or malunion. It leads to a disruption of normal distal radial and ulnar joint function and causes loss of grip strength [22–24].
- Increased radial inclination is seen in Madelung's deformity [25, 26], and it is believed that a steep radial inclination is associated with the development of Kienböck's disease [27].
- The radial inclination is also known as radial angle, radial deviation, or ulnar inclination.

Volar Tilt

- Volar tilt is measured on a conventional lateral radiograph. See Table 6 for the normal values per age category.
- It is defined as the angle between:
  - A line drawn perpendicular to the long axis of the radius (*B*).
  - A tangent line drawn along the slope of the dorsal-to-palmar surface of the radius (*A*) (Fig. 8a, b).

- Volar tilt measurement is used for the assessment of angular displacement. This displacement is often seen in distal radius fractures. Surgeons use volar tilt to plan corrective osteotomies [24, 28].
- Loss of volar tilt results in radial shortening, causing excessive ulnar loading and ulnar-sided wrist pain.
- Volar inclination occurs at the age of 10; hence, volar tilt can be measured from the age of 11. It increases significantly and gradually with age [5].
- Volar tilt is also known as volar angulation, volar inclination, palmar tilt, palmar slope, or palmar inclination.

TABLE 6 Volar tilt age standards measured in degrees (mean) [19]

Age	Male	Female	Combined female and male
8–9	9.23	10.15	9.96
10–11	10.18	10.63	10.43
12–13	12.89	12.89	12.56
14–16	12.35	14.21	13.57

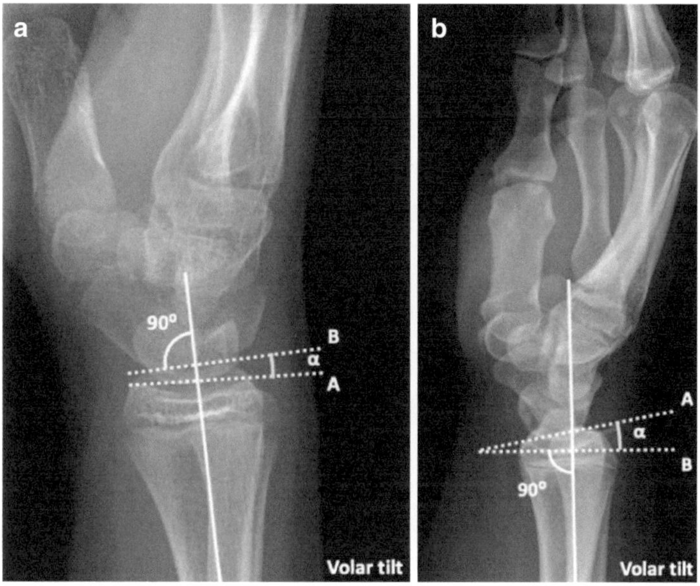

FIGURE 8 Volar tilt measurement. (**a**) 10 years old. (**b**) 15 years old

Cartilage Thickness

- High-frequency ultrasound (US), CT, or MRI can be used in the measurement of cartilage thickness in children. Ultrasound has numerous advantages in the pediatric setting. It is safe and noninvasive, causes no radiation damage, has real-time assessment possibilities, and can be used as a bedside tool, no sedation is needed, and it is easily

TABLE 7 Standards for cartilage thickness measured in millimeters (mean, SD) [32]

Age	Boys	Girls
8 years old	2.00 (1.91–2.09)	1.71 (1.63–1.79)
15 years old	1.18 (1.10–1.26)	0.96 (0.86–1.05)

accepted by children [29]. Additionally, US is more cost- and time-efficient [30] and seems to have high interobserver and intra-observer agreement when measuring cartilage thickness [31].

- The ultrasound measurement of cartilage thickness in the pediatric population is performed in seated position with the wrists laid flat on a table with the palmar side of the hand pointing down. A dorsal longitudinal scan of the articular surfaces of the radial and scaphoid bones side is used to measure cartilage thickness.
- Joint cartilage thickness reduces with age and boys have thicker hyaline cartilage than girls (Table 7) [32, 33].
- In healthy children, no difference in joint cartilage thickness between left and right joints was found [32–34].
- Abnormally, fast cartilage thinning could indicate juvenile idiopathic arthritis, hence the importance of standardized measurements [32, 34–36].

Epiphyseal Overload

- Due to the high demand in high-level sports, young athletes may suffer from stress-related changes of the radial epiphyseal growth plate.
- Epiphyseal overload may be measured on conventional imaging and on MRI:

  - X-ray signs [37]:

    Physeal widening and irregularity.
    Metaphyseal/epiphyseal sclerosis and irregularity.
    Late/advanced stages may show bridging or fusion of the physeal plate.

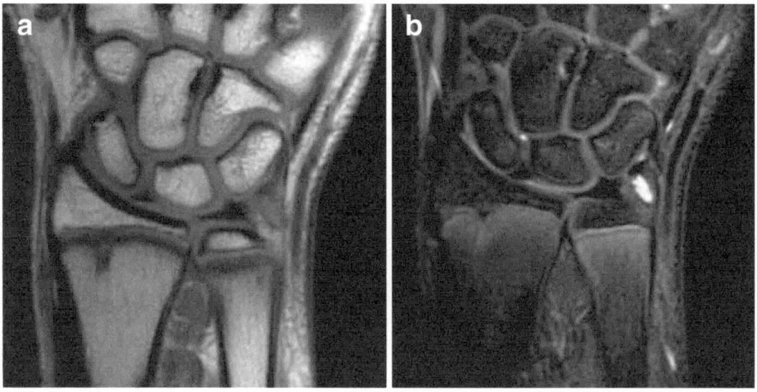

FIGURE 9 Epiphyseal overload. (**a**, **b**) MRI of a 13 year old gymnast with wrist pain. Bone marrow edema is seen in metaphysis of radius and ulna

- MRI signs (Fig. 9a, b):

  Normal distal radial physis: thin physis in the center, and thicker physis peripherally [38].
  Stress-related physeal changes: overall physeal thickening (loss of thin center) especially on the volar side in symptomatic gymnasts (mean increase 30–100% thickening compared to non-gymnasts) [38].
  Increase in water signal fraction up to 35% of 5–10 mm proximal to the physis on T2W-Dixon [39].
  AMPHYS protocol: 12-item scoring tool for grading stress-related changes [13].

- Epiphyseal overload is seen in children with a mean age of 11.7 years (range 6–17 years old; females mean 11.6 years; males mean 12.4 years) [40] with a female predominance (F/M 19:1).
- AMPHYS is the acronym for Amsterdam MRI assessment of the Physis (Table 8).
- Epiphyseal overload is also known as gymnast wrist.

Table 8 AMPHYS scoring tool for epiphyseal overload

	MRI			Grade					
Scoring item	**sequence**	**Radius**	**Ulna**	**0**	**1**	**2**	**3**	**4**	**5**
Epiphysis									
Bone marrow edema									
1.1 Extent	T2 Dixon, PD TSE SPAIR	+	–	No edema	<50% of epiphyseal volume	>50% epiphyseal volume			
1.2 Location					Edema adjacent to physis	Edema not adjacent to physis			
1.3 Signal intensity					1 (min. Signal intensity)	2	3	4	5 (max. Signal intensity)
1.4 Visibility on 3D WATSc	3D WATSc	+	–		Edema not visible		Edema visible		

(continued)

Table 8 (continued)

Scoring item	MRI sequence	Radius	Ulna	Grade 0	1	2	3	4	5
Physis									
2. Thickness	3D WATSc, T2 Dixon, PD TSE			Normal	Increased				
2.1 Compared with MC-1 proximal physis		+	–	Not increased	2× as thick as MC-1	3× as thick as MC-1	4× as thick as MC-1		
3. Signal intensity				Normal signal intensity	1 (min. Signal intensity)	2	3	4	5 (max. Signal intensity)

(continued)

Table 8 (continued)

Scoring item	MRI sequence	Radius	Ulna	Grade 0	1	2	3	4	5
Metaphysis									
4. Physeal border on metaphyseal side	3D WATSc	+	+	Undulating	Slightly irregular	Distinctly irregular			
5. Metaphyseal intrusions				Absent	Present				
5.1 Connection of intrusion with physis				No intrusions	Connected with physis	Not connected with physis			
5.2 Depth of intrusions					<2 mm	>2 mm			
5.3 Signal intensity	T2 Dixon, PD, TSE, 3D WATSc, PD TSE SPAIR			No edema	1 (min. Signal intensity)	2	3	4	5 (max. Signal intensity)

Juvenile Arthritis (JIA)

- Oligo—or polyarthritis has a duration of at least 6 weeks [41, 42].
- There are no specific (angle) measurements specified for JIA, but there are tells/signs which can be assessed on both conventional imaging and MRI.
  - X-rays:

    Soft tissue swelling.
    Osteopenia.
    Loss of joint space.
    Epiphyseal overgrowth ("ballooning").
    Joint subluxation.

  - MRI [43]:

    Joint effusion with or without active synovitis (enhancement in contrast series).
    Dynamic contrast enhancement MRI: steeper slope of contrast enhancement [44].
    Synovial thickening.
    Intra-articular loose bodies ("rice bodies").
    Erosions (osseous and cartilaginous).
    Note that depending on age, young children may need to be sedated to undergo an MRI to ensure optimal image acquisition [45].

- Bony depressions are often mistaken for erosions on an MRI; however, more frequently, they occur naturally during growth in healthy children [46].
- There is a reported peak age 1–4 and 7–10 years old of whom only a proportion tests positive for rheumatoid factor.
- Rice bodies are multiple small loose bodies located inside the joint and have a configuration of rice grains.

Skeletal Age

- To determine the age of a child in addition to the calendar age, the bone age can be assessed to define the biological and structural maturity of pediatric patients. It may be helpful to diagnose growth disorders or to predict the final height of patients with a short stature.
- Skeletal age is defined based on a standard PA radiograph including the wrist (distal radius, ulna, and carpal bones) and the hand (including the carpalia and phalanges) of the nondominant side (see Fig. 10).
  - Greulich and Pyle atlas [47]: reference images per age category and gender to which the radiologist can compare their radiograph to estimate the bone age.
  - Tanner-Whitehouse method [48]: assignment of a score to each bone and gender based on a standard set of bones in different stages of maturation.
  - Three different variations of the Tanner-Whitehouse method exist [49]:
    1) Radius-ulna-short bones: calculation based on 13 bones including the short bones of the fingers (thumb, middle, and little fingers), radius, and ulna.
    2) Carpus: seven carpal bones.
    3) 20-bones method: combination of the two methods above.
- The bone age calculation tools can be used until full ossification of the physes of hand and wrist bones.
- Visibility of ossification centers per age category [50]:
  - Capitate: 1–3 months.
  - Hamate: 2–4 months.
  - Triquetrum: 2–3 years.
  - Lunate: 2–4 years.
  - Scaphoid, trapezium, and trapezoid: 4–6 years.
  - Pisiform: 8–12 years.

- Distal radius: 1 year.
- Distal ulna: 5–6 years.

- The ossification sequence can be remembered by starting with the capitate, moving in an anti-clockward direction to hamate (excluding pisiform bone).

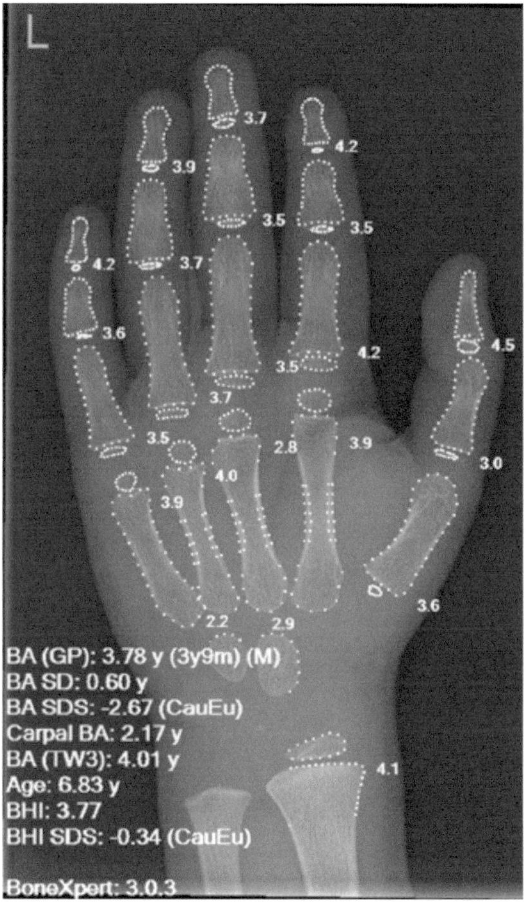

FIGURE 10 6-year-old skeletal bone age calculation based on BoneXpert software

References

1. Slaar A, Bentohami A, Kessels J, Bijlsma TS, van Dijkman BA, Maas M, Wilde JC, Goslings JC, Schep NW. The role of plain radiography in paediatric wrist trauma. Insights Imaging. 2012;3(5):513–7.
2. Williams AA, Lochner HV. Pediatric hand and wrist injuries. Curr Rev Musculoskelet Med. 2013;6(1):18–25.
3. Little JT, Klionsky NB, Chaturvedi A, Soral A, Chaturvedi A. Pediatric distal forearm and wrist injury: an imaging review. Radiographics. 2014;34(2):472–90.
4. Davis KW. Imaging pediatric sports injuries: upper extremity. Radiol Clin North Am. 2010;48(6):1199–211.
5. Sallam AA, Briffa N, Mahmoud SS, Imam MA. Normal wrist development in children and adolescents: a geometrical observational analysis based on plain radiographs. J Pediatr Orthop. 2020;40(9):e860–72.
6. Joyce EA, Farrell T, McMorrow J, Mulholland D, Browne KM, Snow A. Are adult carpal angle measurements applicable to the pediatric population in the trauma setting? Skeletal Radiol. 2018;47(8):1151–6.
7. Schreibman KL, Freeland A, Gilula LA, Yin Y. Imaging of the hand and wrist. Orthop Clin North Am. 1997;28(4):537–82.
8. Alt V, Gasnier J, Sicre G. Injuries of the scapholunate ligament in children. J Pediatr Orthop B. 2004;13(5):326–9.
9. Epner RA, Bowers WH, Guilford WB. Ulnar variance—the effect of wrist positioning and roentgen filming technique. J Hand Surg Am. 1982;7(3):298–305.
10. Hafner R, Poznanski AK, Donovan JM. Ulnar variance in children—standard measurements for evaluation of ulnar shortening in juvenile rheumatoid arthritis, hereditary multiple exostosis and other bone or joint disorders in childhood. Skeletal Radiol. 1989;18(7):513–6.
11. Goldfarb CA, Strauss NL, Wall LB, Calfee RP. Defining ulnar variance in the adolescent wrist: measurement technique and interobserver reliability. J Hand Surg Am. 2011;36(2):272–7.
12. Steyers CM, Blair WF. Measuring ulnar variance: a comparison of techniques. J Hand Surg Am. 1989;14(4):607–12.
13. Kox LS, Kraan RBJ, van Dijke KF, Hemke R, Jens S, de Jonge MC, Oei EHG, Smithuis FF, Terra MP, Maas M. Systematic assessment of the growth plates of the wrist in young gymnasts:

development and validation of the Amsterdam MRI assessment of the physis (AMPHYS) protocol. BMJ Open Sport Exerc Med. 2018;4(1):e000352.
14. Linscheid RL. Biomechanics of the distal radioulnar joint. Clin Orthop Relat Res. 1992;(275):46–55.
15. Shim JI, Im JH, Lee JY, Kang HV, Cho SH. Changes in ulnar variance after a triangular fibrocartilage complex tear. J Wrist Surg. 2019;8(1):30–6.
16. Cerezal L, del Piñal F, Abascal F, García-Valtuille R, Pereda T, Canga A. Imaging findings in ulnar-sided wrist impaction syndromes. Radiographics. 2002;22(1):105–21.
17. De Smet L. Ulnar variance: facts and fiction review article. Acta Orthop Belg. 1994;60(1):1–9.
18. van Leeuwen WF, Oflazoglu K, Menendez ME, Ring D. Negative ulnar variance and Kienböck disease. J Hand Surg Am. 2016;41(2):214–8.
19. Hosseinzadeh P, Olson D, Eads R, Jaglowicz A, Goldfarb CA, Riley SA. Radiologic evaluation of the distal radius indices in early and late childhood. Iowa Orthop J. 2018;38:137–40.
20. Batra S, Gupta A. The effect of fracture-related factors on the functional outcome at 1 year in distal radius fractures. Injury. 2002;33(6):499–502.
21. Földhazy Z, Törnkvist H, Elmstedt E, Andersson G, Hagsten B, Ahrengart L. Long-term outcome of nonsurgically treated distal radius fractures. J Hand Surg Am. 2007;32(9):1374–84.
22. Goldfarb CA, Yin Y, Gilula LA, Fisher AJ, Boyer MI. Wrist fractures: what the clinician wants to know. Radiology. 2001;219(1):11–28.
23. Bessho Y, Nakamura T, Nishiwaki M, Nagura T, Matsumoto M, Nakamura M, Sato K. Effect of decrease in radial inclination of distal radius fractures on distal radioulnar joint stability: a biomechanical study. J Hand Surg Eur. 2018;43(9):967–73.
24. Mann FA, Wilson AJ, Gilula LA. Radiographic evaluation of the wrist: what does the hand surgeon want to know? Radiology. 1992;184(1):15–24.
25. Ali S, Kaplan S, Kaufman T, Fenerty S, Kozin S, Zlotolow DA. Madelung deformity and Madelung-type deformities: a review of the clinical and radiological characteristics. Pediatr Radiol. 2015;45(12):1856–63.
26. Kozin SH, Zlotolow DA. Madelung deformity. J Hand Surg Am. 2015;40(10):2090–8.

27. Mirabello SC, Rosenthal DI, Smith RJ. Correlation of clinical and radiographic findings in Kienböck's disease. J Hand Surg Am. 1987;12(6):1049–54.
28. Arik A, Tanrikulu S, Demiray T, Leblebicioglu G. Radial reference points for measuring palmar tilt and ulnar variance on lateral wrist radiographs. J Hand Surg Asian Pac. 2020;25(1):95–103.
29. Spannow AH, Stenboeg E, Pfeiffer-Jensen M, Fiirgaard B, Haislund M, Ostergaard M, Andersen NT, Herlin T. Ultrasound and MRI measurements of joint cartilage in healthy children: a validation study. Ultraschall Med. 2011;32(Suppl 1):S110–6.
30. Larché MJ, Roth J. Toward standardized ultrasound measurements of cartilage thickness in children. J Rheumatol. 2010;37(12):2445–7.
31. Spannow AH, Pfeiffer-Jensen M, Andersen NT, Stenbøg E, Herlin T. Inter—and intraobserver variation of ultrasonographic cartilage thickness assessments in small and large joints in healthy children. Pediatr Rheumatol Online J. 2009;7:12.
32. Spannow AH, Pfeiffer-Jensen M, Andersen NT, Herlin T, Stenbøg E. Ultrasonographic measurements of joint cartilage thickness in healthy children: age—and sex-related standard reference values. J Rheumatol. 2010;37(12):2595–601.
33. Gau CC, Yao TC, Gan ST, Lin SJ, Yeh KW, Chen LC, Ou LS, Lee WI, Wu CY, Huang JL. Age, gender, height and weight in relation to joint cartilage thickness among school-aged children from ultrasonographic measurement. Pediatr Rheumatol Online J. 2021;19(1):71.
34. Samanta M, Mitra S, Samui PP, Mondal RK, Hazra A, Sabui TK. Evaluation of joint cartilage thickness in healthy children by ultrasound: an experience from a developing nation. Int J Rheum Dis. 2018;21(12):2089–94.
35. Karmazyn B, Bowyer SL, Schmidt KM, Ballinger SH, Buckwalter K, Beam TT, Ying J. US findings of metacarpophalangeal joints in children with idiopathic juvenile arthritis. Pediatr Radiol. 2007;37(5):475–82.
36. Pradsgaard D, Spannow AH, Heuck C, Herlin T. Decreased cartilage thickness in juvenile idiopathic arthritis assessed by ultrasonography. J Rheumatol. 2013;40(9):1596–603.
37. Dobyns JH, Gabel GT. Gymnast's wrist. Hand Clin. 1990;6(3):493–505.
38. Kox LS, Kraan RBJ, Mazzoli V, Mens MA, Kerkhoffs G, Nederveen AJ, Maas M. It's a thin line: development and validation of Dixon MRI-based semi-quantitative assessment of stress-

related bone marrow edema in the wrists of young gymnasts and non-gymnasts. Eur Radiol. 2020;30(3):1534–43.
39. Kraan RBJ, Kox LS, Oostra RJ, Kuijer PPFM, Maas M. The distal radial physis: exploring normal anatomy on MRI enables interpretation of stress related changes in young gymnasts. Eur J Sport Sci. 2020;20(9):1197–205.
40. Heyworth B, Sullivan N, Hart E, Bauer A, Bae D. Gymnast's wrist: a retrospective analysis of descriptive epidemiology, clinical & radiologic features, treatment & outcomes. Orthop J Sports Med. 2019;7:2325967119S2325960006.
41. Marcdante K, Kliegman RM. Nelson essentials of pediatrics. London: Elsevier Health Sciences; 2012.
42. Schwartz MW. The 5 minute pediatric consult. Philadelphia: Lippincott Williams & Wilkins; 2012.
43. Chung C, Coley BD, Martin LC. Rice bodies in juvenile rheumatoid arthritis. Am J Roentgenol. 1998;170(3):698–700.
44. Nusman CM, Lavini C, Hemke R, Caan MWA, Schonenberg-Meinema D, Dolman KM, van Rossum MAJ, van den Berg JM, Kuijpers TW, Maas M. Dynamic contrast-enhanced magnetic resonance imaging of the wrist in children with juvenile idiopathic arthritis. Pediatr Radiol. 2017;47(2):205–13.
45. Rieter JF, De Horatio LT, Nusman CM, Müller LSO, Hemke R, Avenarius DF, Van Rossum MA, Malattia C, Maas M, Rosendahl K. The many shades of enhancement: timing of post-gadolinium images strongly influences the scoring of juvenile idiopathic arthritis wrist involvement on MRI. Pediatr Radiol. 2016;46(11):1562–7.
46. Avenarius DF, Ording Müller LS, Rosendahl K. Erosion or normal variant? 4-year MRI follow-up of the wrists in healthy children. Pediatr Radiol. 2016;46(3):322–30.
47. Greulich WW, Pyle SI. Radiographic atlas of skeletal development of the hand and wrist. Stanford, CA: Stanford University Press; 1959.
48. Tanner JM, Haealy MJR, Cameron N, Goldstein H. Assessment of skeletal maturity and prediction of adult height (TW3 method). London: WB Saunders; 2001.
49. Satoh M. Bone age: assessment methods and clinical applications. Clin Pediatr Endocrinol. 2015;24(4):143–52.
50. Butler P, Mitchell A, Healy JC. Applied radiological anatomy. Cambridge: Cambridge University Press; 2012.

Hand

Saira Haque

Introduction

Significant variations in the sizes of the bones in the hand, and relative portions of the ossified bone, occur in children of different ages. Motion artefact and suboptimal positioning can occur due to difficulty in keeping the hand still, particularly following significant injury. Failure to straighten the digits prevents clear definition of the joint spaces. Parents or caregivers may hold the child's hand flat and help placing items adjacent to the child's hand to obtain optimal imaging.

Skeletal Development of the Hand

- Skeletal maturity occurs in a specific pattern over a predictable timeline which is determined by [1]:
  (a) Development of ossification centres.
  (b) Level of calcium accumulation.
  (c) Bone structure and dimension.

S. Haque (✉)
King's College Hospital NHS Foundation Trust, London, UK
e-mail: saira.haque@nhs.net

P. Simoni, M. P. Aparisi Gómez (eds.), *Essential Measurements in Pediatric Musculoskeletal Imaging*,
https://doi.org/10.1007/978-3-031-17735-4_7

- Rate, duration and amount of growth and maturation vary widely.
- Females, at any age, have advanced bone age compared to males and this is more marked following pubertal onset.
- Epiphyseal region closes approximately 2 years earlier in girls.
- Skeletal maturation lasts longer in males [2].

Carpal Bone Ossification

- Carpal bones are not ossified at birth (Fig. 1).

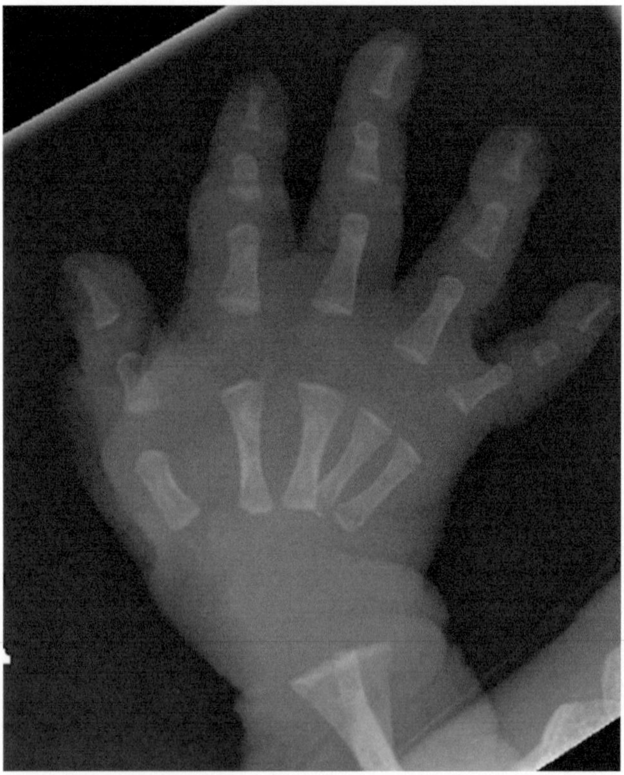

FIGURE 1 Hand radiograph in a 1-month-old neonate demonstrates lack of ossification of the carpal bones

TABLE 1 Lists the mean age of ossification centre appearance in this order: capitate (1), hamate (2), triquetrum (3), lunate (4), trapezium (5), trapezoid (6), scaphoid (7) and pisiform (8)

Carpal bone	
Capitate	1–3 months
Hamate	2–4 months
Triquetrum	2–3 years
Lunate	2–4 years
Trapezium	4–6 years
Trapezoid	4–6 years
Scaphoid	4–6 years
Pisiform	8–12 years

- Significant variation in carpal development due to varying order of appearance, bone fusion or partitioning and development of accessory elements from cartilage [3].
- Approximately one ossification centre appears per year, up to the age of 7 years, except for the pisiform, which as a sesamoid appears during adolescence (Table 1).

Determination of Skeletal Maturity

- The hand and wrist have bones that develop over a clearly defined timeframe and can be easily assessed on a single posterior-anterior radiograph.
- These are key predictors which can aid the determination of skeletal maturity dependent on age [3]:
  1. Infancy (carpal bones and radial epiphyses).
  2. Toddler (number of epiphyses visible in long bones of the hand—Fig. 2).
  3. Prepuberty (ossification centres for phalangeal epiphyses are as wide as metaphyses and increase in thickness—Fig. 3).
  4. Early and mid-puberty (size of phalangeal epiphyses and epiphyses begin to overlap the metaphyses—Fig. 4).

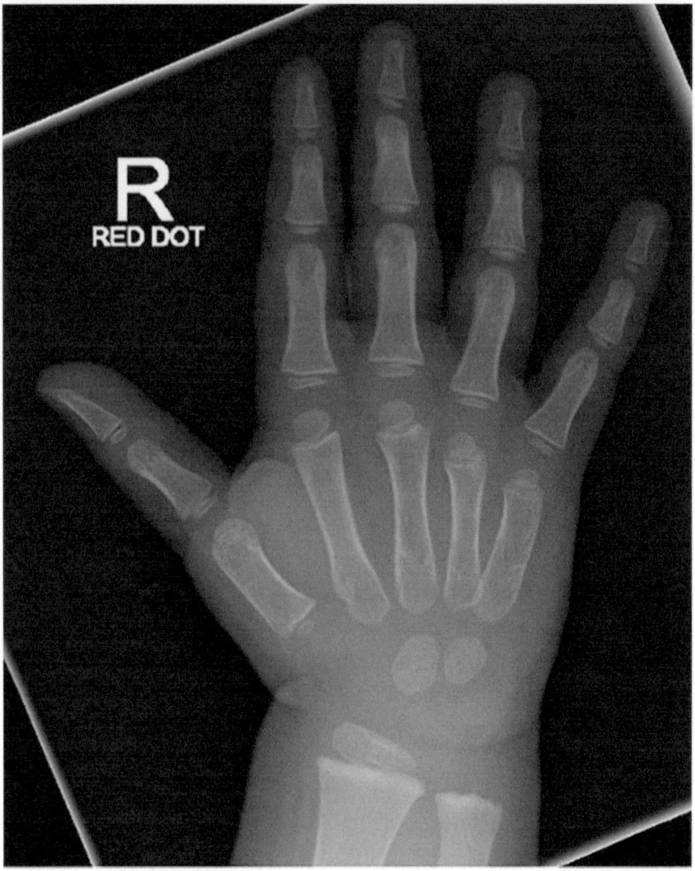

FIGURE 2 Hand radiograph in a 3-year-old male demonstrates ossification of the capitate and hamate

5. Late puberty (fusion of epiphyses to metaphyses in the long bones of the hand in this order: distal phalanges [first], metacarpals [second], proximal phalanges [third] and finally fusion of middle phalanges).
6. Post-puberty (extent of epiphyseal fusion of radius and ulna).

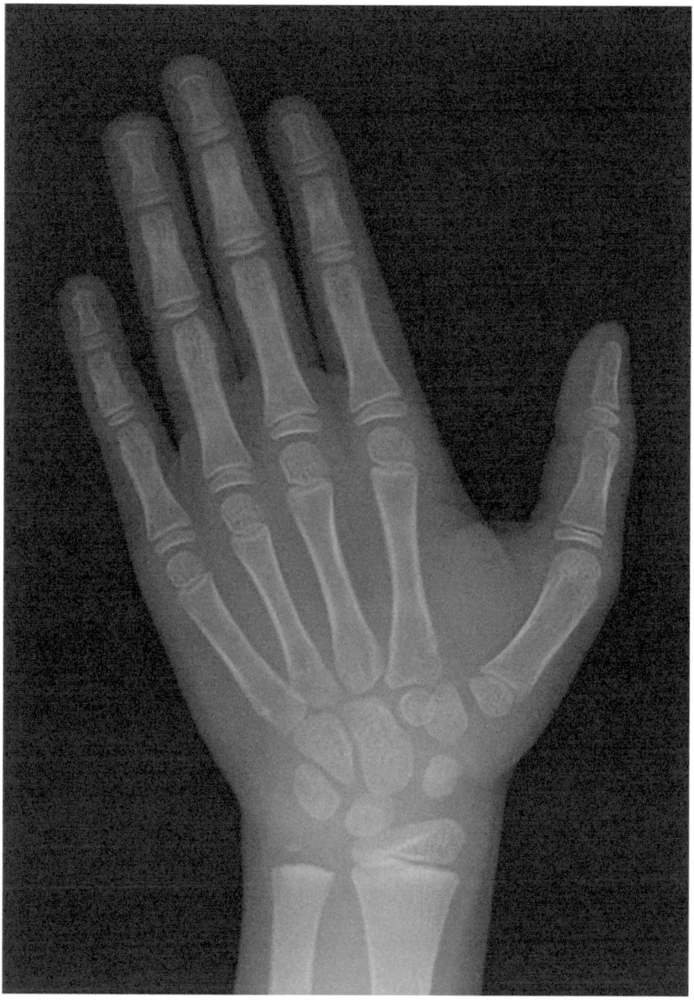

FIGURE 3 Hand radiograph in a 5-year-old male demonstrates ossification centres for phalangeal epiphyses are becoming as wide as the metaphyses

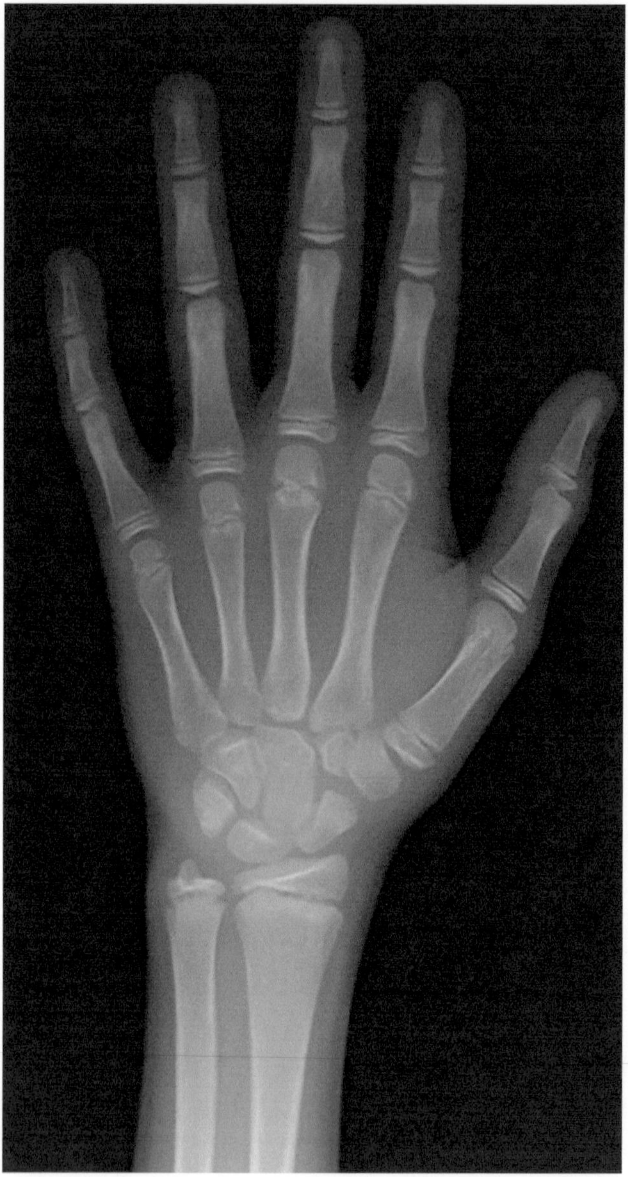

FIGURE 4 Normal radiograph in a 13-year-old female showing that the phalangeal epiphyses begin to overlap the metaphyses

- Most common technique used to determine the level of bone maturation of the nondominant hand (in years) is Greulich and Pyle (G&P).
- Chronological age (in years) is determined from the child's birth date.
- Observers are more likely to interpret the radiograph as normal when chronologic age is known than when it is not.
- Ultrasound can be used to assess endochondral ossification and is of particular use to assess growth by assessment of distal radial and ulna epiphysis, using gender- and ethnicity-based algorithms [4].
- Magnetic resonance (MR) imaging is useful in growth assessment as it allows accurate assessment of the tubular and carpal bones.
- Epiphyseal cartilage, morphological appearance and size of the epiphyses, physeal structure/closure (bone bridges), zone of provisional calcification and progression of ossification are well assessed using MR imaging [5].

Carpal Angle

- Defined as the angle between:
  (a) Line from proximal surface of the scaphoid and lunate.
  (b) Line through the proximal triquetrum and lunate.

  Normal value = 130°.
  Increased (>139°): trisomy 21 and Pfeiffer syndrome.
  Decreased (<118°): Hurler's syndrome, Morquio syndrome and Madelung deformity (Fig. 5).

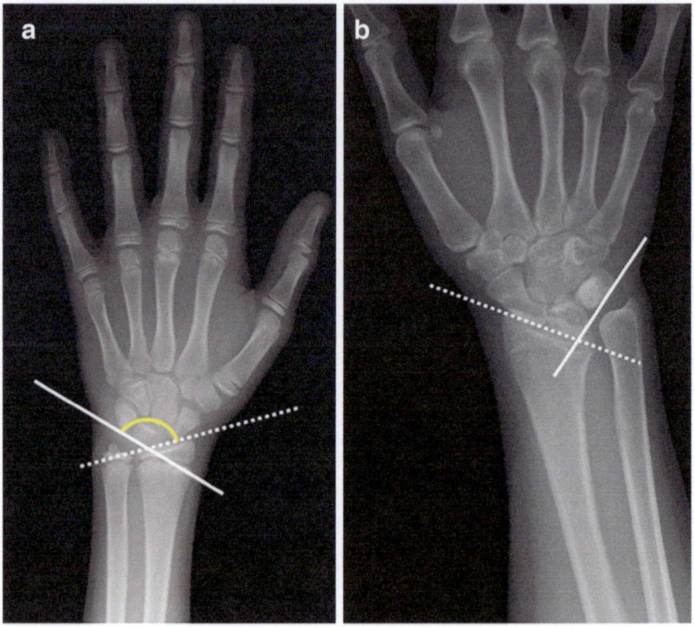

FIGURE 5 (**a**) Normal carpal angle, measured between the line from the proximal surface of the scaphoid and lunate (white dotted line) to the line through the proximal triquetrum and lunate (white bold line). (**b**) Reduced carpal angle in a case of Madelung deformity

Carpal Height

- Defined by the distance between the midpoint of the distal radial epiphysis ossification center and the proximal end of the third metacarpal [6].
- Useful in assessing congenital malformations, particularly when the carpus is not fully ossified.
- Carpal height increases as the child gets older.

- Carpal height ratio in children is similar to that seen in adults [7].
- The normal range of the carpal height ratio (calculated by dividing the carpal height by the length of the third metacarpal) is between 0.51 and 0.57 [8].
- Shortening of the carpus: multiple epiphyseal dysplasia, otopalatodigital syndromes, Turner syndrome, arthrogryposis and juvenile idiopathic arthritis (Figs. 6 and 7).

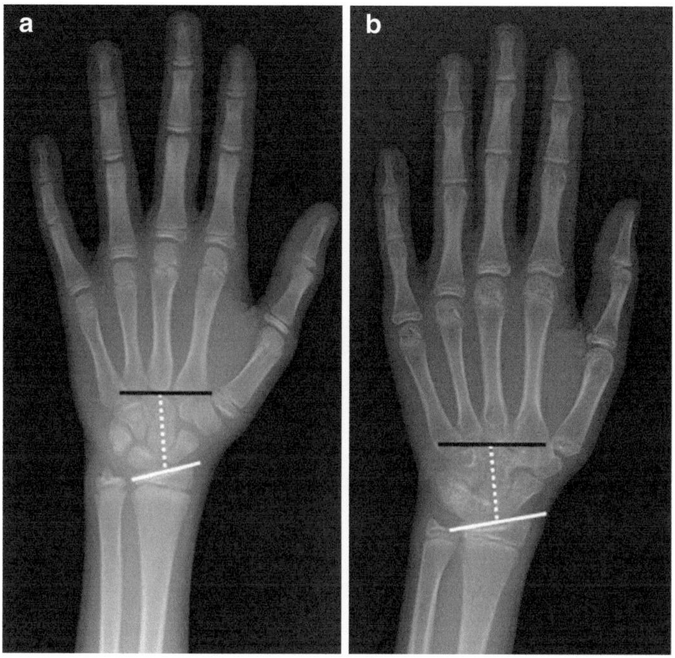

FIGURE 6 (**a**) The carpal height (white dotted line) is the distance between the midpoint of the distal radial epiphyseal ossification center (white line) and proximal end of the third metacarpal (black line). This is reduced due to carpal crowding in a 13-year-old (**b**)

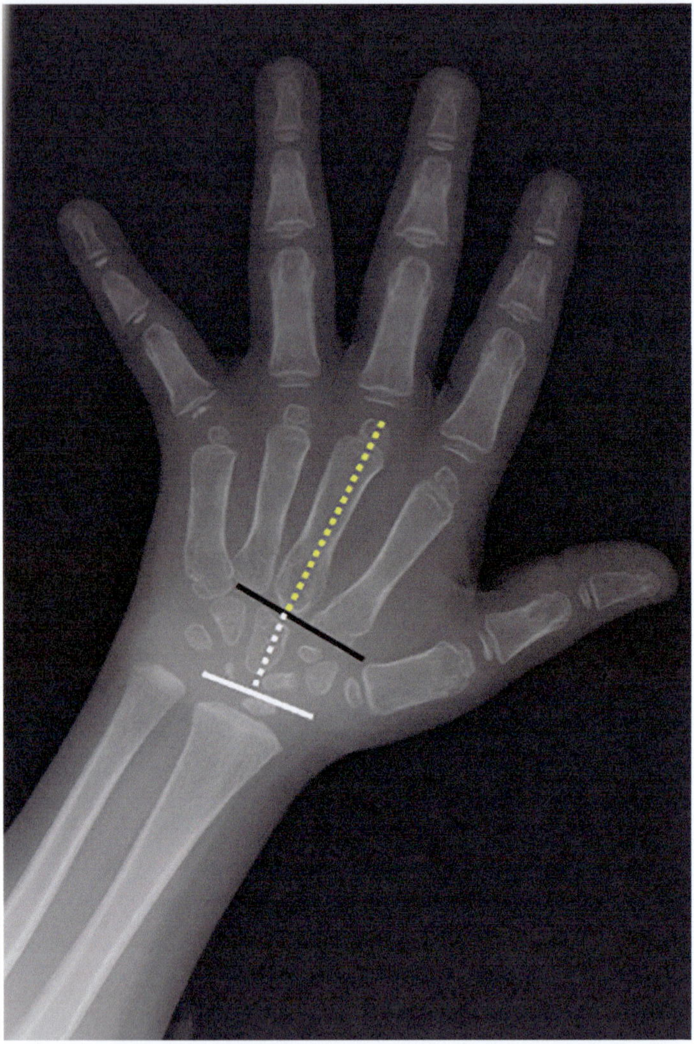

FIGURE 7 7-year-old with spondyloepiphyseal dysplasia. Reduction in carpal height due to hypoplasia of the carpal bones; the carpal height ratio has been calculated by dividing the carpal height (white dotted line) by the length of the third metacarpal (yellow dotted line). The midpoint of the distal radial epiphyseal ossification center is indicated by the white line and the proximal end of the third metacarpal depicted by the black line

Scapholunate Distance

- Scapholunate distance of less than or equal to 2 mm is used to assess for soft tissue injuries in adults [9].
- In younger children, this distance is normally wider due to the larger chondral component of the scaphoid and lunate, and this decreases with age [10].
- Boys have a longer distance than girls due to earlier skeletal maturity and develop adult values from 12 years of age (Figs. 8 and 9).
- Mean Scapholunate Distance According to Age [11]
  6 Years: 7–9 mm
  7 Years: 6–8 mm
  8 Years: 5.5–7.5 mm
  9 Years: 5–6.5 mm
  10 Years: 4.5–6 mm
  11 Years: 4–5 mm
  12 Years: 3.5–4.5 mm

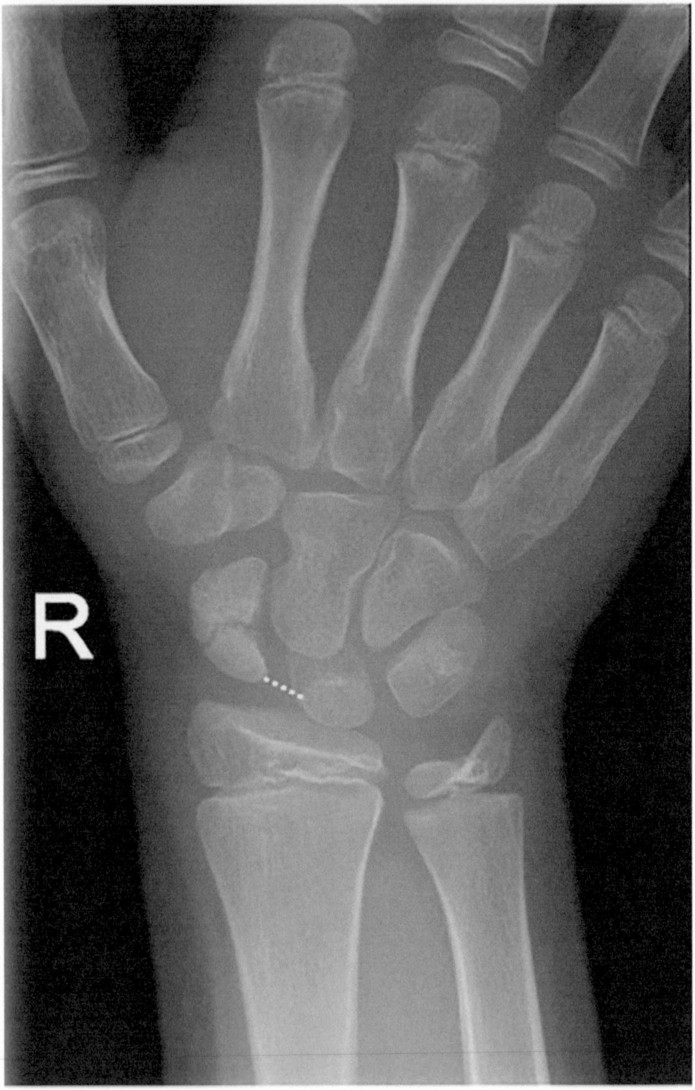

FIGURE 8 12-year-old male with a scaphoid waist fracture and widening of the scapholunate distance (dotted yellow line) secondary to a scapholunate ligamentous injury

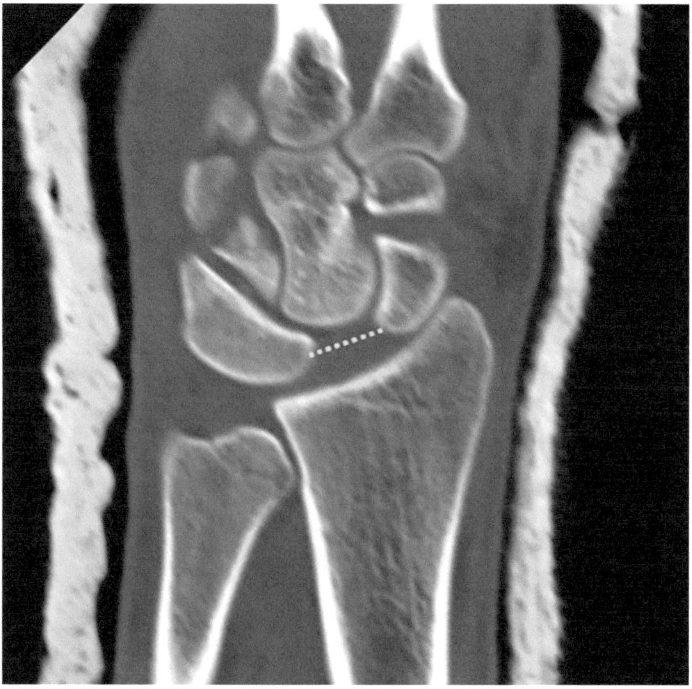

FIGURE 9 Coronal CT image of a 15-year-old male with significant widening of the scapholunate distance (dotted yellow line) measuring 10 mm; incidental note of lunotriquetral coalition

Carpal Instability

- Scapholunate and capitolunate angles can be used on lateral radiographs or sagittal imaging to assess carpal instability.
- This is possible when the carpal bones are ossified appropriately, for example, when the proximal and distal poles of the scaphoid are discernible [12].
- Capitolunate angle: angle between the long axis of the capitate and the mid-axis of the lunate.
- Mean capitolunate angle is 11° (SD ± 7°).

- This angle is increased in dorsal intercalated segment instability and volar intercalated segment instability; the scapholunate angle is used to differentiate between these two entities.
- Scapholunate angle: angle between line drawn through the axis of the scaphoid and lunate.
- Mean scapholunate angle is 47° (SD ± 8), and if this angle is >80°and the lunate is extended, features are suggestive of dorsal intercalated segmental instability.

Metacarpal Index

- This is a measure of the slenderness of the metacarpals.
- Metacarpal index increases from lower values in early childhood to adult range by 10 to 11 years in normal children [13].
- Ratio of mean length to mean width of second to fifth metacarpals, measured at their midpoints.
- A second method involves dividing the sum of the lengths by the sum of the widths of the metacarpals.
- Normal metacarpal index <7–9 (Fig. 10) but in arachnodactyly it is >8.5 (metacarpals are longer and thinner than normal).
- Arachnodactyly is associated with Marfan syndrome, osteogenesis imperfecta, dystrophia myotonica, homocystinuria and Ehlers-Danlos syndrome [14].
- It is important to note that the metacarpal index is a poor discriminator of patients with tall stature or clinical signs of arachnodactyly; these patients should still be examined for additional signs of Marfan syndrome or other inherited disorders of connective tissue.

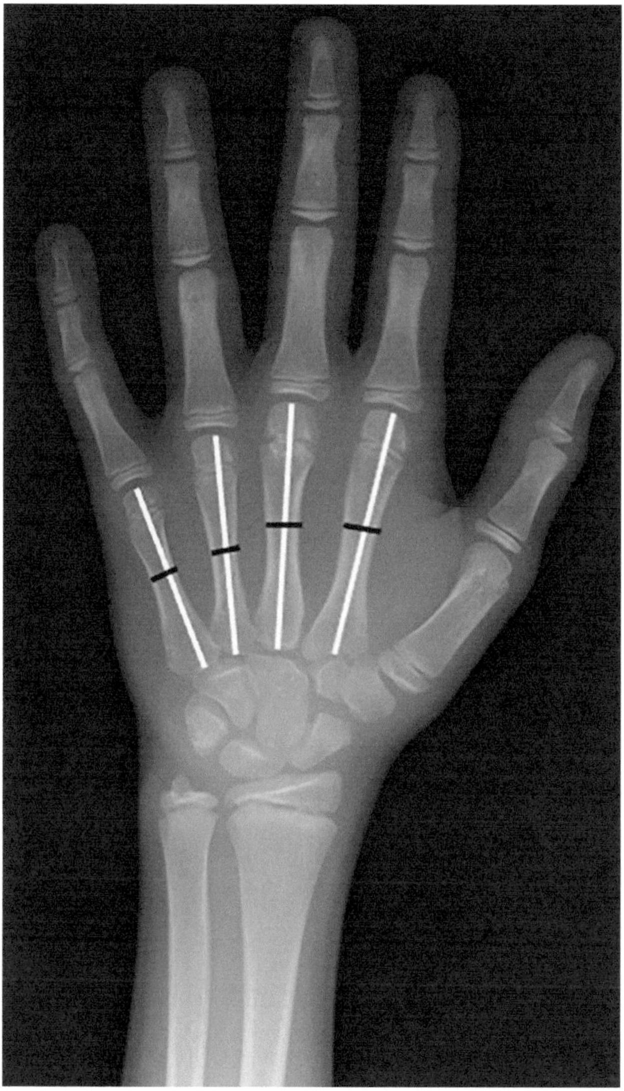

FIGURE 10 Metacarpal index in a 13-year-old girl, within the normal range (value was 7). The metacarpal index is determined by dividing the length of each of the last four metacarpals (white lines) by the width of the midpoint (black lines) and averaging the values

Metacarpal Sign

- Assesses the lateral three metacarpals by drawing a tangential line along the distal fifth and fourth metacarpals.
- Normally, this passes distal to the head of the third metacarpal, but if this intersects the third metacarpal, the fourth metacarpal is considered short.
- Can be seen as normal variant, Turner syndrome, pseudohyperparathyroidism, acrodysostosis and occasionally homocystinuria (Fig. 11).
- This sign is negative if all metacarpals are short or if there is greater shortening of the third metacarpal than the fourth metacarpal [15].

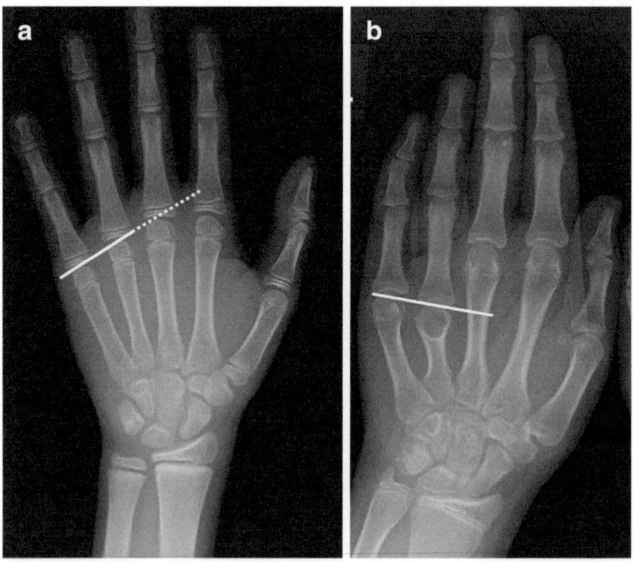

FIGURE 11 In image (**a**), a tangential line drawn along distal fifth and fourth metacarpals (white line) passes distal to head of the third metacarpal (dotted line). In image (**b**), the tangential line (white line) drawn along distal fifth and fourth metacarpals extends to the mid-shaft of the third metacarpal in a patient with Turner syndrome

Brachydactyly

- Congenital: shortened hands due to absence or rudimentary development of metacarpals and/phalanges; inherited (usually dominant trait) but can be part of a syndrome (Fig. 12).
- PA view of the hands is the first-line investigation.
- Brachyphalangy (abnormal short phalanges), brachybasophalangia (proximal), brachymesophalangia (middle) and brachytelephalangia (distal).

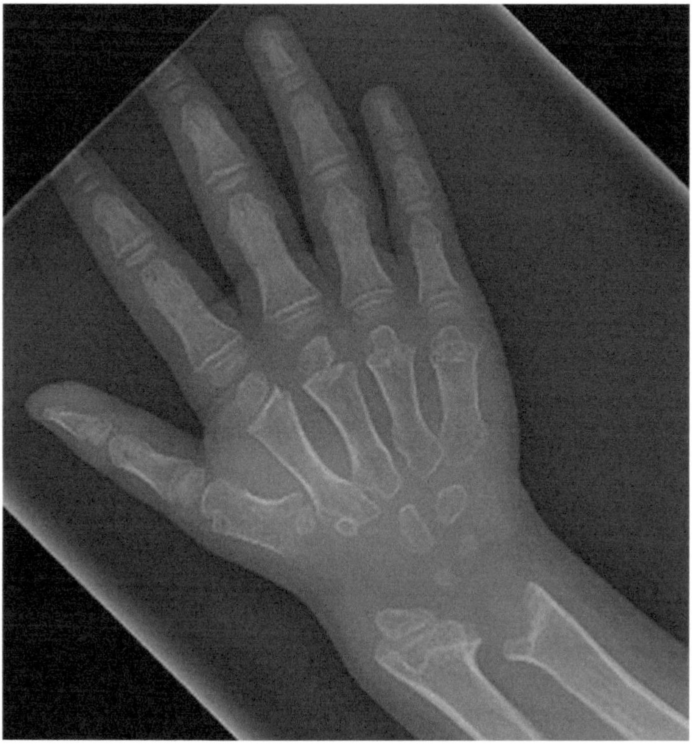

FIGURE 12 This image of a 5-year-old patient with mucopolysaccharidosis (MPS) type IV demonstrates brachydactyly with widened and shortened tubular bones, shortening of the metacarpals, pointing of the second through fifth metacarpals and irregular carpal bones

- Most used index of digit length: ratio of middle finger (cm) to hand length (cm)—measured with hand open from fingerprint to the principal crease where finger joins the palm and the palm joins the wrist; middle finger length (50th centile): 5 cm (4 years), 6 cm (8 years), 7 cm (12 years) and 8 cm (16 years) [16].

Joint Fluid

- Even small effusions (1 mm) can be detected in the hand joints with an interobserver agreement of 79% using ultrasound [17].
- Dorsal recesses are measured using ultrasound in a mid-sagittal view.
- The hand is kept in a neutral position as flexion leads to reduction or disappearance of the fluid (Fig. 13).
- Mean depth of radiocarpal recess = 0.4 mm (SD 0.5, range 0–2.9) [18].
- Mean depth of midcarpal recess = 0.5 mm (SD 0.6, range 0–2.4).

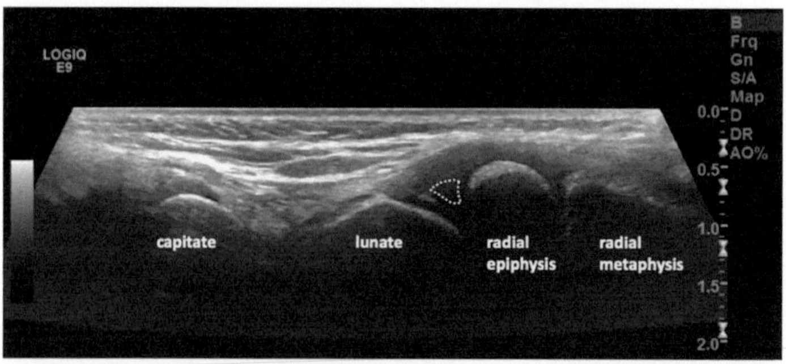

FIGURE 13 Dorsal recess (outlined in dotted line) of the radiocarpal joint has been measured using ultrasound in the mid-sagittal view

- No differences according to sex, but increasing depth of the recesses by age.
- One or more vessels are seen in 8% of the radiocarpal and 4% of the midcarpal recesses (Fig. 14).
- There is a considerable variation in normal synovial thickness, up to 5 mm [19] (Fig. 15).

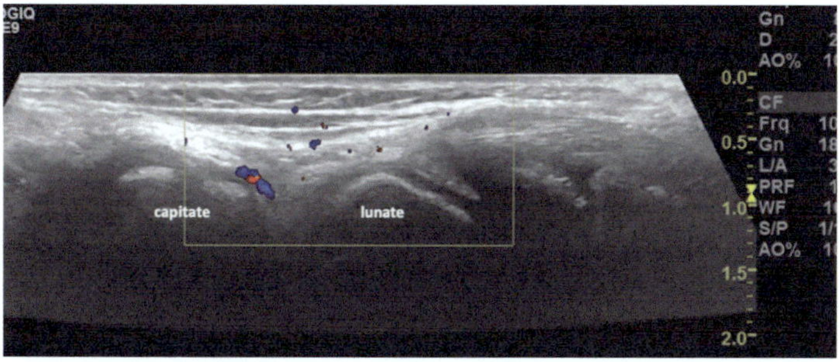

FIGURE 14 Mid-sagittal view of the midcarpal joint using ultrasound demonstrates a normal vessel

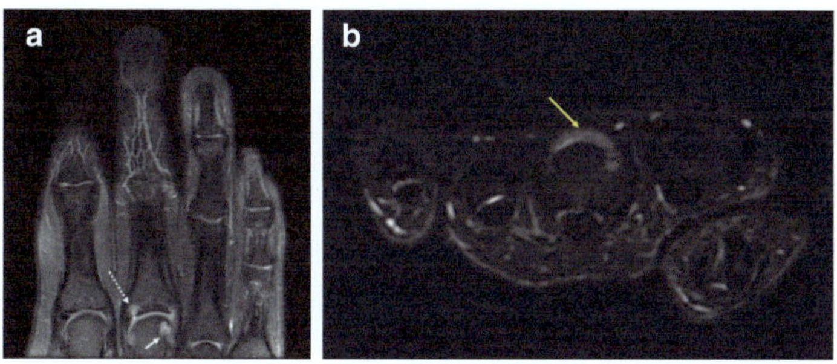

FIGURE 15 This coronal (**a**) and axial (**b**) STIR MR images in an 11-year-old girl demonstrate joint fluid in the middle finger metacarpal joint, synovial proliferation (yellow arrow in the axial view), and erosions at the metacarpal head (white arrow in the coronal view) and proximal phalanx of the middle finger (dotted arrow in the coronal view)

Tendon Pathology

- There is a strong linear relationship between tendon thickness and age, with the tendon thickness increasing with age.
- Minimal fluid (0.3 mm) can be seen in the tendon sheaths of children; a hypoechoic rim can be detected around the finger tendon sheath particularly on the palmar aspect of the metacarpal [20].
- Ultrasound is superior to MRI in depicting dynamic pathology and allowing comparison with the opposite side (Fig. 16).

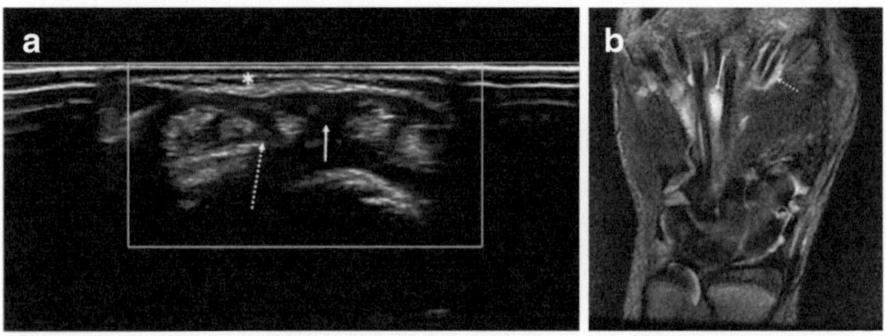

FIGURE 16 4-year-old who presented with hand swelling. Transverse ultrasound image (**a**), with colour Doppler flow, demonstrates thickening of the synovial sheath (8 mm thickness) of the extensor digitorum tendons (white arrow), increased vascularity (dotted arrow) and peritendinous subcutaneous oedema (asterisk). Coronal STIR image on MR (**b**) performed subsequently also demonstrates fluid (yellow arrow) and synovial thickening (dotted yellow arrow) surrounding the extensor digitorum tendons

Paediatric Trigger Thumb

- Results in abnormal flexion at the interphalangeal joint due to thickening of the flexor pollicis longus tendon (secondary to abnormal synovial proliferation, collagen degeneration).
- Triggering occurs when the cross-sectional area of the flexor pollicis longus exceeds the cross-sectional area demarcated by the A1 pulley (Fig. 17); unilateral triggering and a trigger ratio (maximal cross-sectional area of involved FPL to uninvolved FPL) <1.5 are at risk for developing triggering bilaterally [21, 22].

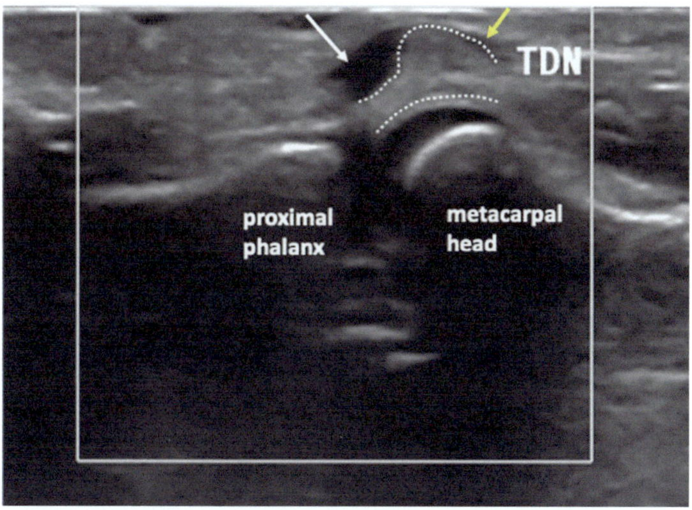

FIGURE 17 Longitudinal ultrasound image in an 11-month-old demonstrates the metacarpal joint of the thumb with developmental mismatch between the thickened FPL tendon (yellow arrow) and the area under the A1 pulley (white arrow)

Carpal Tunnel

- Carpal tunnel syndrome is best assessed by looking at the median nerve echogenicity, proximal to the retinaculum flexorum, and by identifying the site of greatest nerve enlargement.
- Wrist-to-forearm ratio of proximal and distal cross-sectional area measurement of the median nerve is also helpful for assessment [23] (Fig. 18). Wrist-to-forearm ratio in normal circumstances approaches 1. In carpal tunnel syndrome, there is thickening of the nerve at the wrist.
- Prominent signs of carpal tunnel syndrome include hypoechogenicity or a wrist-to-forearm ratio >1.5.
- Moderate signs of carpal tunnel syndrome include hypoechogenicity and a wrist-to-forearm ratio >2.

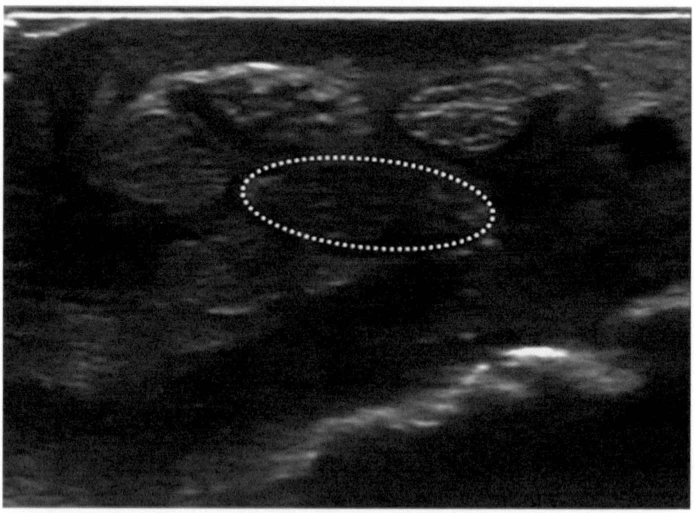

FIGURE 18 Transverse ultrasound image of the right median nerve (outlined) at the level of the carpal tunnel, proximal to the retinaculum flexorum, in a 9-year-old female, demonstrates enlargement and reduced echogenicity consistent with carpal tunnel syndrome

References

1. Tanner JM, Whitehouse RH. Growth at adolescence. 2nd ed. Springfield, IL: Blackwell Scientific; 1962.
2. Mora S, Boechat MI, Pietka E, Huang HK, Gilsanz V. Skeletal age determinations in children of European and African descent: applicability of the Greulich and Pyle standards. Pediatr Res. 2001;50:624–8. https://doi.org/10.1203/00006450-200111000-00015.
3. Cavallo F, Mohn A, Chiarelli F, Giannini C. Evaluation of bone age in children: a mini-review. Front Pediatr. 2021;9:580314. https://doi.org/10.3389/fped.2021.580314.
4. Mentzel HJ, Vilser C, Eulenstein M, et al. Assessment of skeletal age at the wrist in children with a new ultrasound device. Pediatr Radiol. 2005;35:429–33. https://doi.org/10.1007/s00247-004-1385-3.
5. Tomei E, Sartori A, Nissman D, Al Ansari N, Battisti S, Rubini A, Stagnitti A, Martino M, Marini M, Barbato E, Semelka RC. Value of MRI of the hand and the wrist in evaluation of bone age: preliminary results. J Magn Reson Imaging. 2014;39(5):1198–205. https://doi.org/10.1002/jmri.24286. PMID: 25006631
6. Poznanski AK, Hernandez RJ, Guire KE, Bereza UL, Garn SM. Carpal length in children—a useful measurement in the diagnosis of rheumatoid arthritis and some concenital malformation syndromes. Radiology. 1978;129(3):661–8. PMID: 725041. https://doi.org/10.1148/129.3.661.
7. Sallam AA, Briffa N, Mahmoud SS, Imam MA. Normal wrist development in children and adolescents: a geometrical observational analysis based on plain radiographs. J Pediatr Orthop. 2020;40(9):e860–72. PMID: 32404657. https://doi.org/10.1097/BPO.0000000000001584.
8. Youm Y, McMurthy RY, Flatt AE, Gillespie TE. Kinematics of the wrist. I. an experimental study of radial-ulnar deviation and flexion-extension. J Bone Joint Surg Am. 1978;60(4):423–31. PMID: 670263.
9. Okan N, Caboğlu F, Mertoğlu T, Durakbaşa O, Görgeç M. Cocuklarda the measurement of wrist kinematics in children 4 to 16 years old and the comparison of the scapholunate distance with adult values. Acta Orthop Traumatol Turc. 2004;38(1):30–3. PMID: 15054295.

10. Kaawach W, Ecklund K, Di Canzio J, Zurakowski D, Waters PM. Normal ranges of scapholunate distance in children 6 to 14 years old. J Pediatr Orthop. 2001;21(4):464–7.
11. Leicht P, Mikkelsen B, Larsen CF. Scapholunate distance in children. Acta Radiol. 1996;37(5):625–6.
12. Joyce EA, Farrell T, McMorrow J, et al. Are adult carpal angle measurements applicable to the pediatric population in the trauma setting? Skeletal Radiol. 2018;47:1151–6.
13. Rand TC, Edwards DK, Bay CA, et al. The metacarpal index in normal children. Pediatr Radiol. 1980;9:31–2. https://doi.org/10.1007/BF00973966.
14. Nelle M, Tröger J, Rupprath G, Bettendorf M. Metacarpal index in Marfan's syndrome and in constitutional tall stature. Arch Dis Child. 1994;70(2):149–50. https://doi.org/10.1136/adc.70.2.149.
15. Poznanski AK. Useful measurements in the evaluation of hand radiographs. Hand Clin. 1991;7(1):21–36. PMID: 2037636.
16. Normogram can be found in the Appendix of Jones, ed. Smith's recognizable patterns of human malformation, 5th ed. Philadelphia: Saunders; 1997. [Sivan Y, Merlob P, Reisner SH. Upper Limb Standards in Newborns. Am J Dis Child. 1983;137(9):829–32]. https://doi.org/10.1001/archpedi.1983.02140350007003.
17. Szkudlarek M, Court-Payen M, Jacobsen S, Klarlund M, Thomsen HS, Ostergaard M. Interobserver agreement in ultrasonography of the finger and toe joints in rheumatoid arthritis. Arthritis Rheum. 2003;48:955–62. https://doi.org/10.1002/art.10877.
18. Rosendahl K, Bruserud IS, Oehme N, et al. Normative ultrasound references for the paediatric wrist; dorsal soft tissues. RMD Open. 2018;4:e000642. https://doi.org/10.1136/rmdopen-2017-000642.
19. Smith MD. The normal synovium. Open Rheumatol. 2017;12:63.
20. Collado P, Naredo E, Calvo C, Crespo M. Assessment of the joint recesses and tendon sheaths in healthy children by high-resolution B-mode and power Doppler sonography. Clin Exp Rheumatol. 2007;25(6):915–21. PMID: 18173930.
21. Verma M, Craig CL, DiPietro MA, Crawford J, VanderHave KL, Farley FA, Caird MS. Serial ultrasound evaluation of pediatric trigger thumb. J Pediatr Orthop. 2013;33(3):309–13. PMID: 23482269. https://doi.org/10.1097/BPO.0b013e318287f728.

22. Kim J, Gong HS, Seok HS, Choi YH, Oh S, Baek GH. Quantitative measurements of the cross-sectional configuration of the flexor pollicis longus tendon using ultrasonography in patients with pediatric trigger thumb. J Hand Surg Am. 2018;43(3):284.e1–7. Epub 2017 Sep 19. https://doi.org/10.1016/j.jhsa.2017.08.011.
23. Descatha A, Huard L, Aubert F, Barbato B, Gorand O, Chastang JF. Meta-analysis on the performance of sonography for the diagnosis of carpal tunnel syndrome. Semin Arthritis Rheum. 2012;41(6):914–22.

Hip and Pelvis

Nele Herregods, Jacob Jaremko, and Lennart Jans

Introduction

The hip of the child is not a miniature adult hip. In immature hips, the structures that later will result in the neck, head, and greater trochanter are initially cartilaginous and progressively ossify (Fig. 1a). The greater trochanter and the femoral head are completely ossified by the age of 12. The femoral head and greater trochanter share the same growth plate that closes only after puberty. The blood perfusion of the femoral head in children depends solely on an arterial anastomotic network in the posterior region of the femoral neck. There is no flow to the

N. Herregods (✉)
Department of Radiology and Nuclear Medicine, Ghent University Hospital, Ghent, Belgium
e-mail: nele.herregods@uzgent.be

J. Jaremko
Department of Radiology, University of Alberta, Edmonton, AB, Canada

L. Jans
Department of Radiology and Nuclear Medicine, Ghent University Hospital, Ghent, Belgium

P. Simoni, M. P. Aparisi Gómez (eds.), *Essential Measurements in Pediatric Musculoskeletal Imaging*,
https://doi.org/10.1007/978-3-031-17735-4_8

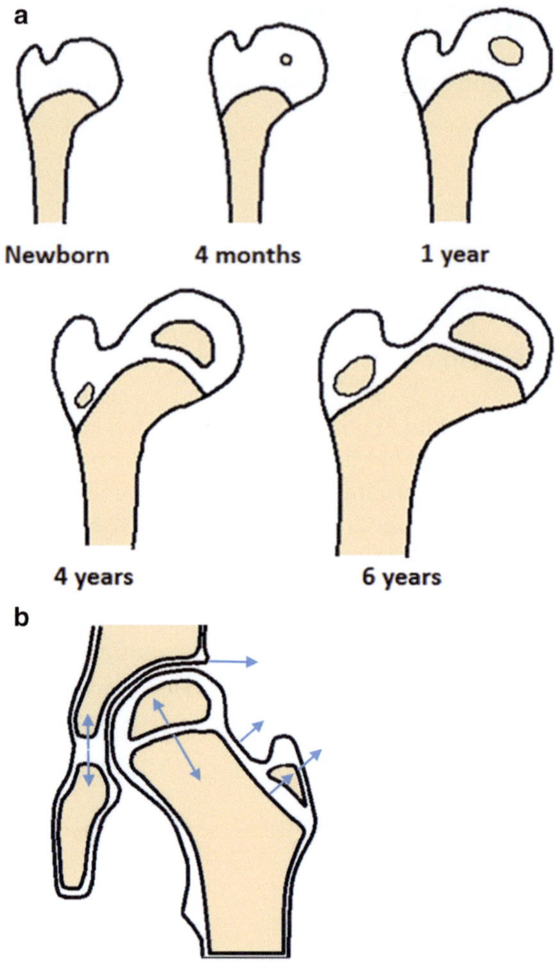

Figure 1 (**a**) Schematic representation of the growing human proximal femur, showing the femoral head and greater trochanter ossification centers at different ages. (**b**) Growth of the hip: The acetabulum grows in depth and width from the triradiate cartilage and by apposition from the edge. A secondary ossification center at the edge of the acetabulum appears in the early second decade, known as os acetabuli. The greater trochanter enlarges by physeal growth up to 8 years of age, after which growth is appositional. Acetabulum and greater trochanter growth is physeal and appositional. (With permission from Herregods et al. [1])

femoral head due to the presence of a growth plate. Only in children below 18 months, there are transphyseal vessels to the epiphysis. There is growth in the transition area from the head to the femoral neck (growth cartilage), responsible for normal growth of the femoral head and neck lengthening, growth cartilage in the greater trochanter, and the triradiate growth cartilage of the acetabulum that grows in depth and width so as to maintain its sphericity and concavity and hold the femoral head in joint (Fig. 1b). Lesion or trauma of these regions may predispose to severe anomalies in the development of the femoral head or deformities of the acetabulum [1, 2].

Developmental Dysplasia (DDH)

- In children >5–6 months of age, radiography is indicated because progressing ossification of the femoral head prevents adequate evaluation with US [3].
- For infants <4–5 months of age, ultrasound (US) is still the imaging modality of choice [4, 5].
- Several lines and angles are used to diagnose and further characterize DDH: Hilgenreiner's, Perkin's, and Shenton's line, and the acetabular and center-edge angle [1, 6].
- A second AP radiograph of the pelvis with the thighs in abduction, flexion, and external rotation (i.e., frog-leg lateral projection) is performed to determine whether a displaced or subluxed hip is reducible [7].

Hip Acetabular Angle

- Measured on anteroposterior (AP) radiograph of the hips in a neutral position.
- Formed by a horizontal line connecting both triradiate cartilages (Hilgenreiner's line) and a second line which extends along the acetabular roofs (Fig. 2).
- In adolescents where the triradiate cartilages are fused and therefore inapparent, the inferior margin of the pelvic teardrop is used instead.
- Normal values for different ages are shown in Table 1 [8].

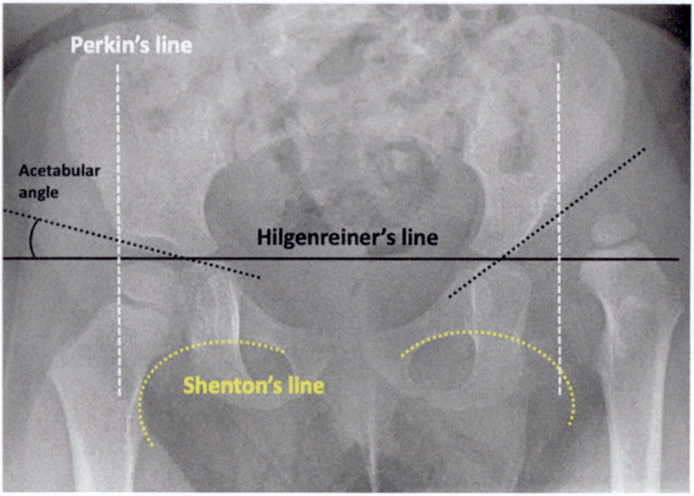

FIGURE 2 Anteroposterior radiograph showing Hilgenreiner's, Perkin's, and Shenton's lines, and the acetabular angle. There is developmental dysplasia of the left hip with increased acetabular angle, a shallow acetabulum, and dislocation. Note delayed ossification of the left femoral head epiphysis. The right hip joint is normal. (Permission from Herregods et al. [1])

TABLE 1 Normal values of acetabular angles for different ages and sexes [8]

Age	Acetabular angle females	Acetabular angle males
Newborn	28.8° ± 4.8°	26.4° ± 4.4°
3 months old	25° ± 3.5°	22° ± 4°
6 months old	23.2° ± 4.0°	20.3° ± 3.7°
1 year old	21.2° ± 3.8°	19.8° ± 3.6°
>2 years old	18° ± 4°	19° ± 3.6°

- Perkin's line is a line drawn perpendicular to Hilgenreiner's line, intersecting the lateral most aspect of the acetabular roof. The upper femoral epiphysis should be seen in the inferomedial quadrant, below Hilgenreiner's line, and medial to Perkin's line.
- If the nucleus of the femoral head is not visible because it is not ossified yet, the femoral metaphysis should be used.

Acetabular Coverage of the Femoral Head

The percent of the acetabular head coverage is calculated by dividing the distance between the acetabular floor line and a horizontal line extending from the iliac bone (d), by the distance between the acetabular floor and joint capsule line/femoral head diameter (D) multiplied by 100. A cutoff value of 50% is advocated (Fig. 3a) [9].

US Alpha-Beta Angle

- The American College of Radiology recommends that a standard US examination includes static images in two orthogonal planes and dynamic imaging.
- A coronal view in the "Graf standard plane" with three essential landmarks: the inferior border of the ilium, osseous acetabular roof, and labrum (Fig. 3a); transverse views of the flexed hip with and without stress and dynamic assessment to determine the position and stability of the femoral head, with a technique similar to the clinical Barlow examination.
- The Graf α and β angles are measured on a coronal image (Fig. 3a, b): the osseous acetabular roof angle (α angle) and acetabular cartilaginous (labrum) angle (β angle) [10, 11].

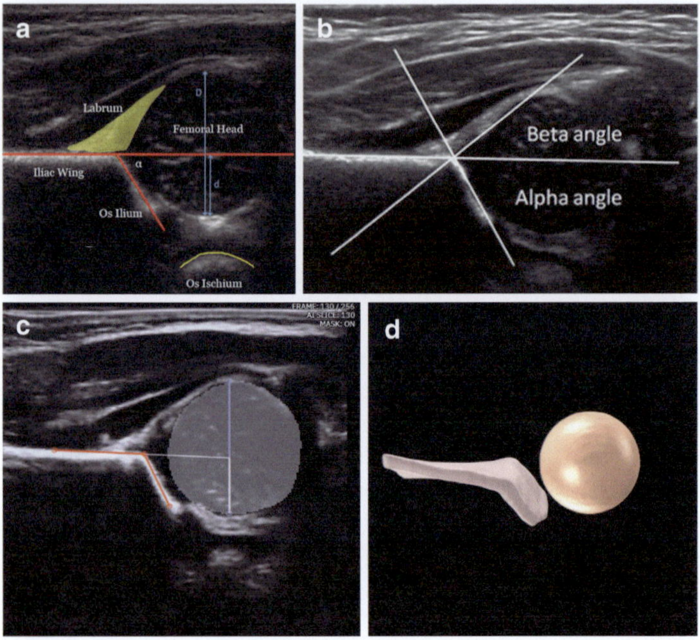

FIGURE 3 (**a**) Coronal ultrasound image in the "Graf standard plane" through the mid-hip joint with flat iliac wing, round femoral head, os ilium and os ischium visible, showing the measurement of the Graf α angle and acetabular coverage (d/D) and (**b**) Graf α (alpha) and β (beta) angles. (**c**) Automated identification of acetabulum and femoral head (segmentation) by artificial intelligence from 3D ultrasound, with (**d**) the corresponding 3D shape model. (Credit: Medo.ai)

- The modified Graf grading classification (four types listed in Table 2) is based on the α angle and degree of acetabular roof coverage [3].
- Three-dimensional (3D) US is an emerging imaging modality for infant's hips. 3D shape indices can be generated to diagnose hip dysplasia more reliably and offer further insight into the 3D aspects of the deformity (Fig. 3c, d) [12].

TABLE 2 Modified Graf classification scale (Permission from Herregods et al. [1])

Graf type	Description	α and β angle
Type 1	Normal, mature hip with more than 50% acetabular roof coverage	α angle ≥60° β angle <55°
Type 2a	Physiologic immaturity at younger than 3 months	α angle 50–59°
Type 2b	Immature at age 3 months or older	α angle 50–59°
Type 2c	Extremely deficient bony acetabulum; femoral head is concentric but not stable	α angle 43–49° β angle <77°
Type 2d	Femoral head is grossly subluxed and labrum is everted, increasing β angle	α angle difficult to measure but is approximately 43–49° β angle >77°
Type 3	Dislocated femoral head with shallow acetabulum	α angle <43°
Type 4	Dislocated femoral head with severely shallow, dysplastic acetabulum and inverted labrum	

- A scan protocol in which the whole hip joint is imaged by cine-sweep or 3D ultrasound improves reliability for non-expert users [13]. This type of scan is also amenable to automated analysis by artificial intelligence (AI). An AI app called Medo Hip using this approach has been cleared by US-FDA (https://www.medo.ai/aria-hip). In the future, population screening for hip dysplasia could be done by portable ultrasound performed by nurses and interpreted automatically by AI.

Medial Joint Space (Teardrop Distance)

- The medial joint space is used to determine lateral displacement of the femoral head on radiographs.
- It is defined as the distance measured from the medial edge of the femoral head ossification nucleus (where it is broadest just above the growth plate) to the adjacent acetabular wall.
- When the ossification nucleus is absent or asymmetric, measurement is made from the femoral neck metaphysis just below the growth plate.
- This measurement is best made on the frog-lateral projection [14].
- Normal range from 6 months to 11 years = 5–12 mm.
- In side-to-side comparison, the difference between measurements of the medial joint space should be less than 1.5 mm.

Shenton's Line

- Shenton's line is an imaginary curved line drawn along the inferior border of the superior pubic ramus (superior border of the obturator foramen) and along the inferomedial border of the neck of femur (Fig. 2).
- This line should be continuous and smooth.
- Interruption of the Shenton's line can indicate DDH or fractured neck of femur.

Perkin's Line

- Perkin's line is a line drawn perpendicular to Hilgenreiner's line, intersecting the most lateral aspect of the acetabular roof (Fig. 2).
- The upper femoral epiphysis should be seen in the inferomedial quadrant: it should lie below Hilgenreiner's line, and medial to Perkin's line.

- If the nucleus of the femoral head is not visible because it is not ossified yet, the femoral metaphysis should be used as reference.
- Lateral displacement of the femoral head occurs in DDH.

Lateral Center-Edge Angle (Wiberg)

- The lateral center-edge angle is a radiographic measurement to evaluate lateral coverage of the femoral head by the acetabulum.
- This angle is calculated on AP pelvic radiographs by drawing a best-fit circle for the inferior and medial margins of the femoral head. The angle is then measured between two lines drawn from the center of the circle, one running vertically along the longitudinal axis of the pelvis and the other one tangential to the lateral margin of the acetabular rim (Fig. 4).

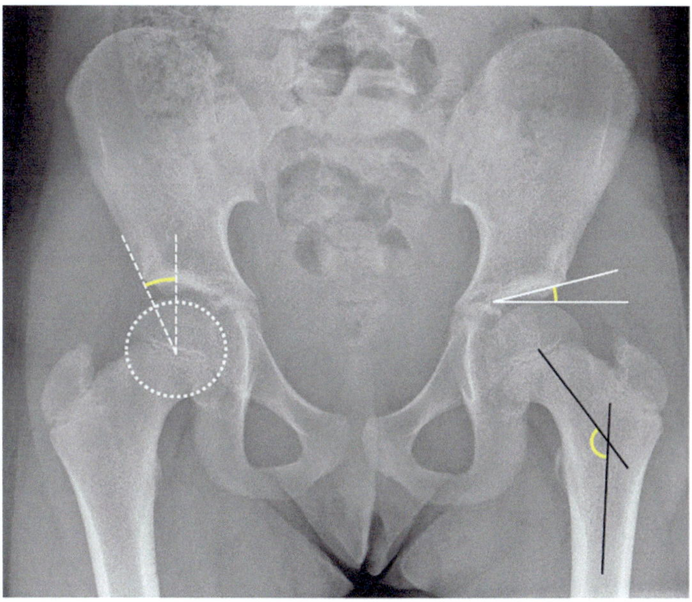

FIGURE 4 Anteroposterior radiograph showing the lateral center-edge angle (Wiberg) (dashed white lines), Tönnis angle (bold white lines), and femoral head-neck-shaft angle (bold black lines)

- Reference lateral center edge angles are 25° for children aged 0 (neonates) to 8 years and 32° for children older than 8 years to aged 18 years [15].
- Values <20° indicate acetabular dysplasia, between 20° and 25°: borderline acetabular dysplasia.
- Values of >39°indicate overcoverage (pincer-type impingement).

Vertical-Center-Anterior Angle

- The vertical-center-anterior angle is measured on a false profile view (Lequesne profile).
- This angle is used to evaluate anterior coverage of the femoral head and is formed by a vertical line through the femoral head center and a line connecting the femoral head center and anterior edge of the acetabular roof (Fig. 5).
- An angle of 20°–25° indicates borderline dysplasia, and an angle of less than 20° indicates dysplasia [6].

Tönnis Angle

- The Tönnis angle is used to measure the acetabular surface and is formed by a horizontal line and a tangential line extending from the medial to lateral sclerotic edges of the acetabular roof (Fig. 4) [16].
- A Tönnis angle greater than 13° is abnormal.

Pubofemoral Distance

- Pubofemoral distance (PFD) is a reproducible measurement of hip instability; it is an easy sonographic screening test to avoid late diagnosis of developmental dysplasia of the hip.

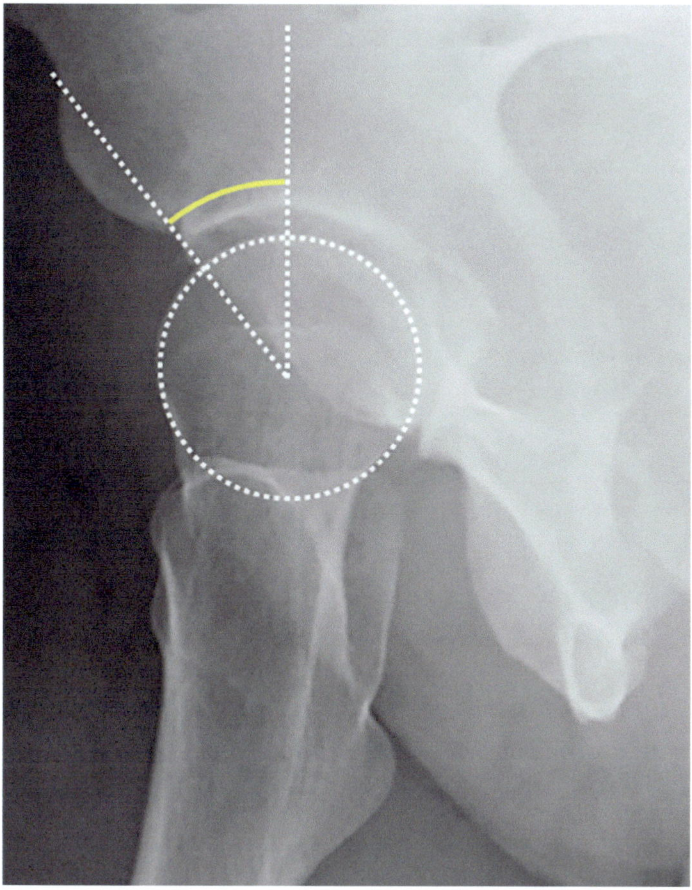

Figure 5 Image illustrating the vertical-center-anterior angle in the false profile view (Lequesne profile)

- PFD is measured between the medial margin of the epiphysis and the pubic bone (Fig. 6).
- PFD >6 mm (at the age of 1 month) or a difference >1.5 mm should lead to expert referral [17].

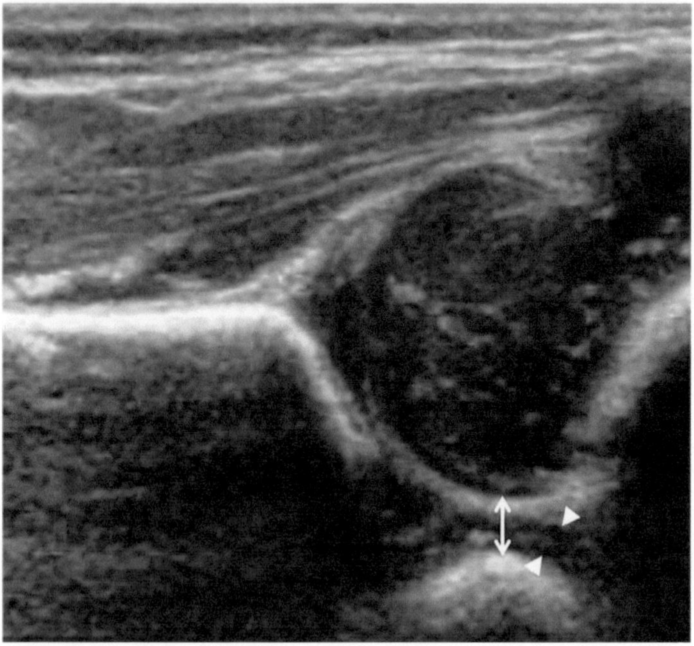

FIGURE 6 Ultrasound image illustrating the measurement of the pubofemoral distance (double-headed arrow) between the pubic bone and the femoral head. Arrowheads indicate the pubic cartilage thickness

Femoral Head-Neck-Shaft Angle

- The femoral head-neck-shaft angle is formed by the intersection of the femoral neck axis and femoral long axis (Fig. 4).
- The normal femoral neck-shaft angle ranges between 120° and 135°, and it decreases from 150° in infants to 120° in adults [18].
- In coxa vara, the angle is decreased to <120°, and in coxa valga, the angle is increased to >135° (Fig. 7).
- External rotation of the femur should be avoided during patient positioning because as little as 7° of external rota-

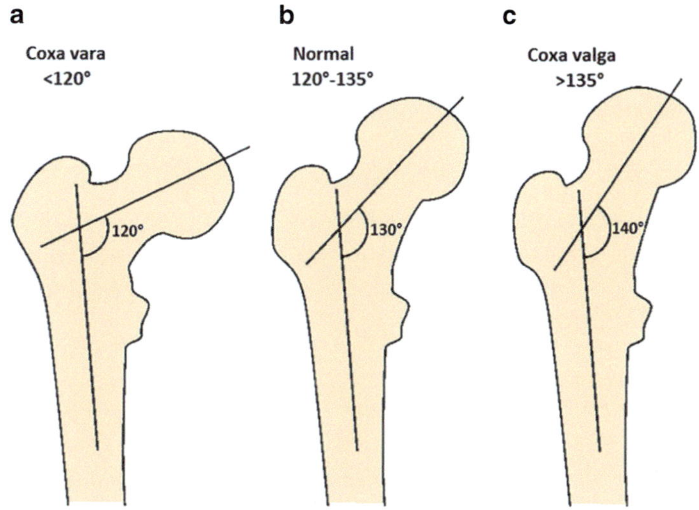

FIGURE 7 Femoral neck-shaft angle (black lines) in (**a**) coxa vara, (**b**) normal hip, and (**c**) coxa valga. (Permission from Herregods et al. [1])

tion may result in a >10° change in the measurement of the neck-shaft angle [19].

Slipped Capital Femoral Epiphysis (SCFE)

Klein's Line

- The Klein's line is a parallel line that is drawn along the lateral border of the femoral neck and intersects a small portion of the femoral epiphysis (FE) in normal hips.
- Hips with medial displacement of the FE lack this intersection (Fig. 8a). A 2-mm or greater difference in the epiphyseal width lateral to the Klein line between the hips strengthens the diagnosis of SCFE, with a sensitivity of 79% [20].

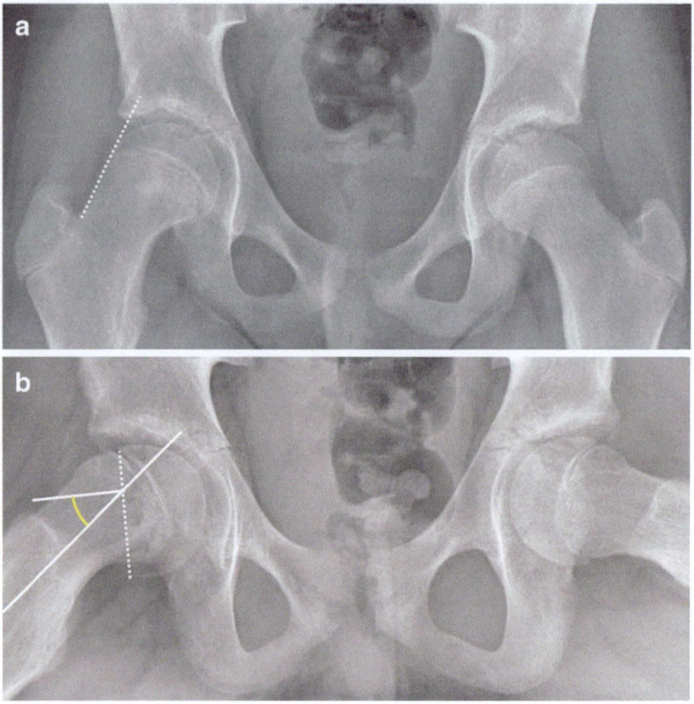

FIGURE 8 (**a**) Anteroposterior radiographs showing the Klein line and (**b**) Southwick SCFE measurement in the frog-leg lateral view

Southwick's Method

- The Southwick's method measures angular epiphyseal displacement by using the epiphyseal shaft angle on a frog-leg lateral radiograph.
- The epiphyseal shaft angle is formed between a line that is perpendicular to a line that connects the anterior and posterior margins of the FE and a line along the axis of the femoral shaft (Fig. 8b).

- Subtraction of the epiphyseal shaft angle value on the unaffected side from that on the affected side yields the epiphyseal slippage grade; in cases of bilateral slippage, a 12° angle is used as a normal reference.
- The severity of the slippage is classified as mild (<30° difference between angles), moderate (30°–50° difference), or severe (>50° difference).
- Three-dimensional imaging should be considered for patients with limited hip flexion or external hip rotation [21].
- MRI may depict very early physeal changes without evidence of slippage during the "preslip" stage, when radiographs and CT scans show normal findings [22].

Femoroacetabular Impingement (FAI)

- There are two primary forms of FAI: cam type, which is a proximal femur abnormality, and pincer type, which is an acetabular component abnormality.
- For initial evaluation of the acetabulum, plain radiographs of the pelvis are recommended and an additional view of the femoral neck such as Dunn's views, cross-table lateral, frog-leg lateral, or Meyer lateral for the assessment of the femoral head-neck junction [23].
- At anteroposterior radiography, characteristic cam impingement findings are sphericity and abnormal contour of the femoral head and femoral neck junction [6].
- Cross-table lateral or Dunn's radiographic view of the hip or oblique axial (CT or MR) images along the femoral neck are used for evaluation of the extent of the cam deformity by measuring the anterior offset distance and the α angle.
- For pincer-type FAI, lateral center-edge angle, Tönnis angle, ilioischial line, crossover sign, posterior wall sign, and acetabular anteversion can be measured or observed.

Anterior Offset Distance

- The anterior offset is the distance from two parallel lines to the femoral neck axis measured on an axial view of the femur. One line is traced tangential to the anterior contour of the femoral head. The second line is traced to the point where the femoral head becomes aspherical (is no longer spherical), at the same point of the α angle (Fig. 9).
- An anterior offset distance shorter than 10 mm suggests FAI.

Alpha Angle

- The α angle is formed by the femoral neck axis and a line connecting the femoral head center to the point where the femoral head is no longer spherical (Fig. 9).
- An α angle of greater than 55°–60° is abnormal.

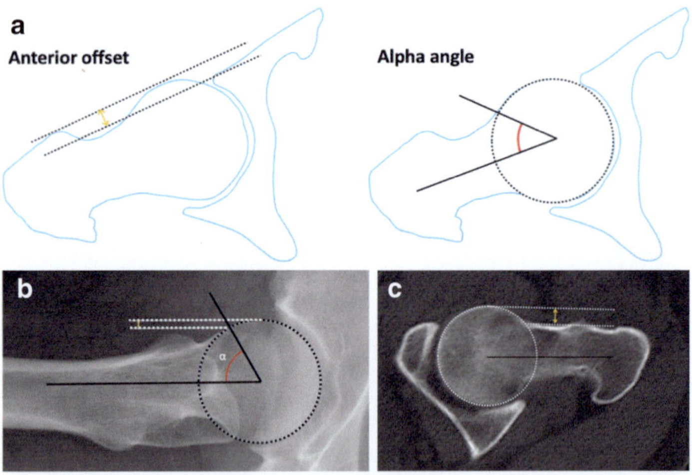

FIGURE 9 (**a**) Schematic drawings, (**b**) axial radiographic view, and (**c**) axial CT view of the proximal femur illustrating the anterior offset distance (orange double-headed arrows on **a**, **b** and **c**) and the alpha angle (black lines, angle depicted in red in **a** and **b**)

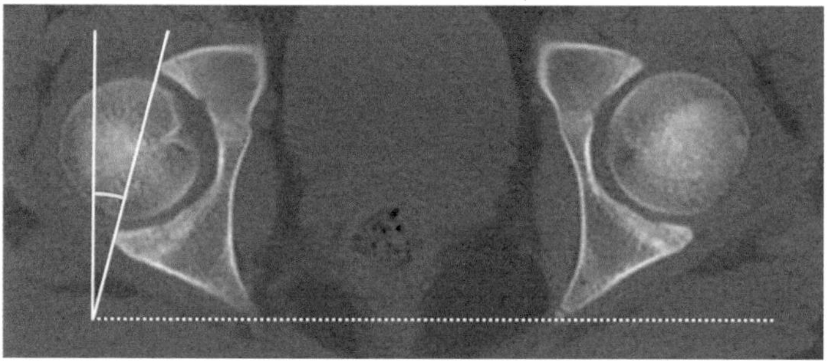

FIGURE 10 Measurements of acetabular anteversion

Acetabular Anteversion

- Axial CT image is used for measuring acetabular anteversion at the level of the femoral head center. Acetabular anteversion refers to the angulation of the line between the anterior and posterior acetabular margins and a line perpendicular to either the intercapital line or a horizontal line between the posterior pelvic margins at the sciatic notch level (Anda's method) (Fig. 10).

Lines: Arcuate/Acetabular Roof-Teardrop

- The arcuate line marks the border between the corpus and ala of the iliac bone. It runs inferior, anterior, and medial to the articular surface of the area corresponding to the acetabulum (Fig. 11).
- The iliopectineal, or arcuate line is a landmark for the anterior column. The ilioischial line is a landmark for the posterior column. The acetabular roofline and "teardrop" are a landmark for the medial portion of the acetabulum.
- The acetabular teardrop (U-figure, "Köhler's teardrop") represents the projection of a bony ridge along the floor of the acetabular fossa (Fig. 11).
- An increased space of >11 mm increased distance between the pelvic teardrop and the femoral head or >2 mm in comparison to the contralateral hip indicates hip joint effusion [24].

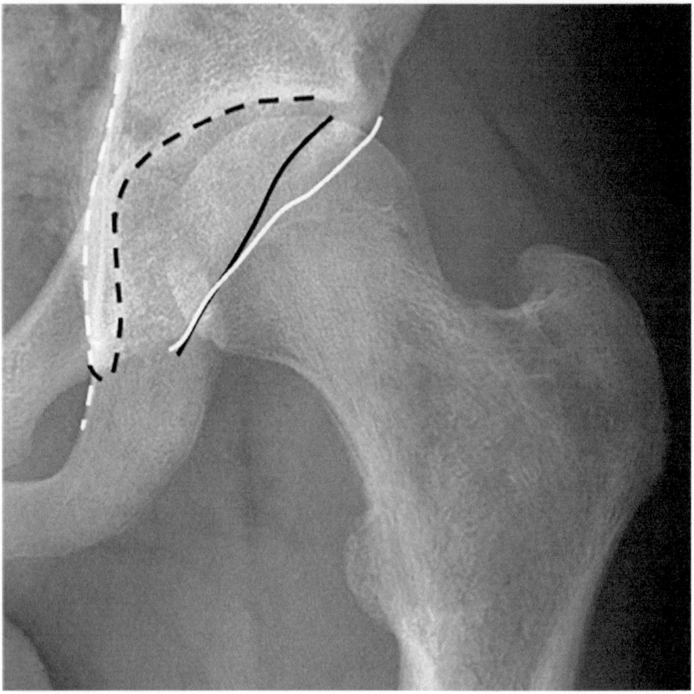

Figure 11 Anteroposterior radiograph showing the ilioischial line (dashed white line), the acetabular roof line (dashed black line), and acetabular "teardrop." The bold white line is the posterior rim of the acetabulum, and the bold black line is the anterior acetabular rim

Pelvic Tilt

- The pelvic tilt is easiest measured on a lateral view of the pelvis. Pelvic tilt is measured from the angle between a vertical line and the line joining the mid point of the upper sacral end plate and the hip axis (Fig. 12).
- Normal values for boys are 6.5 ± 7.5° (range: −10.2 to 30.0). Normal values for girls are 8.5 ± 8.3° (range: −17.2 to 29.7). Pelvic tilt tends to increase during growth.
- Numerous methods have been described for the estimation of pelvic tilt on AP pelvis radiograph. The most reliable estimator that has been described is the sacrococcygeal

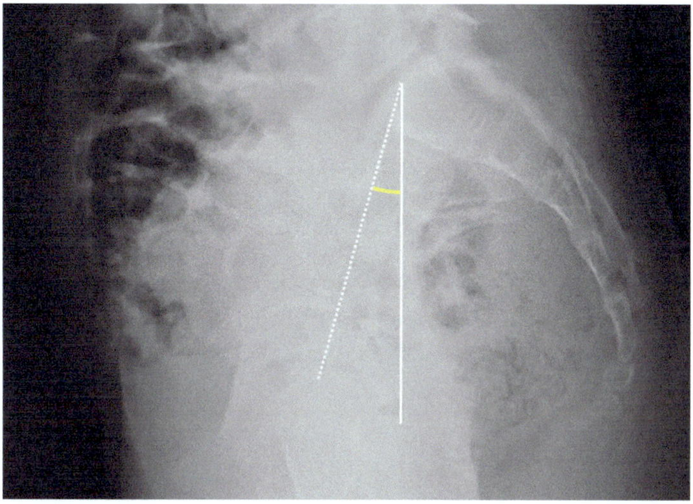

FIGURE 12 Lateral pelvic radiograph illustrating measurement of pelvic tilt. This is the angle between the vertical (bold white line) and a line joining the mid point of the upper sacral endplate and the hip axis (dotted white line)

joint to symphysis pubis distance; this is the distance between the midportion of the sacrococcygeal joint and the upper border of the public symphysis. The normal value is about 32 mm in men and 47 mm in women.

- Variation in the pelvic tilt on radiographs influences the acetabular measurements such as the acetabular index, lateral center-edge angle, crossover sign, Tönnis angle, or acetabular coverage [25–28].

Pubic Symphyseal Width

- The transverse width of the symphysis pubis using a focus-film distance of 1 m is measured to the nearest tenth of a millimetre.
- Normal values gradually decrease from 7.4 + −1.3 mm aged 0–6 months to 5.4 mm aged 16 years [9].

References

1. Herregods N, Vanhoenacker FM, Jaremko JL, Jans L. Update on pediatric hip imaging. Semin Muskuloskeletal Radiol. 2017;21:561–81. https://doi.org/10.1055/s-0037-1606134.
2. Lee MC, Eberson CP. Growth and development of the child's hip. Orthop Clin North Am. 2006;37(02):119–32. https://doi.org/10.1016/j.ocl.2005.12.001.
3. Starr V, Ha BY. Imaging update on developmental dysplasia of the hip with the role of MRI. AJR Am J Roentgenol. 2014;203(06):1324–35.
4. Bracken J, Tran T, Ditchfield M. Developmental dysplasia of the hip: controversies and current concepts. J Paediatr Child Health. 2012;48(11):963–72; quiz 972–973.
5. Bracken J, Ditchfield M. Ultrasonography in developmental dysplasia of the hip: what have we learned? Pediatr Radiol. 2012;42(12):1418–31.
6. Silva MS, Fernandes ARC, Cardoso FN, Longo CH, Aihara AY. Radiography, CT, and MRI of hip and lower limb disorders in children and adolescents. Radiographics. 2019;39:779–94. https://doi.org/10.1148/rg.2019180101.
7. Grissom LE. The pelvis and hip: congenital and developmental conditions. In: Stein-Wexler R, Wootton-Gorges S, Ozonoff M, editors. Pediatric orthopedic imaging. Berlin: Springer; 2015. p. 273–318.
8. Caffey in Ozonoff MB. Pediatric orthopedic radiology. Philadelphia: W.B. Saunders; 1992. p. 181.
9. Keats T, Sistrom S. Atlas of radiologic measurement. 7th ed. Philadelphia, PA: Mosby; 2001.
10. American Institute of Ultrasound in Medicine. AIUM practice guideline for the performance of an ultrasound examination for detection and assessment of developmental dysplasia of the hip. J Ultrasound Med. 2013;32(07):1307–17.
11. Graf R. Classification of hip joint dysplasia by means of sonography. Arch Orthop Trauma Surg. 1984;102(04):248–55.
12. Jaremko JL, Mabee M, Swami VG, Jamieson L, Chow K, Thompson RB. Potential for change in US diagnosis of hip dysplasia solely caused by changes in probe orientation: patterns of alpha-angle variation revealed by using three-dimensional US. Radiology. 2014;273(03):870–8.

13. Mostofi E, Chahal B, Zonoobi D, et al. Reliability of 2D and 3D ultrasound for infant hip dysplasia in the hands of novice users. Eur Radiol. 2019;29(3):1489–95. https://doi.org/10.1007/s00330-018-5699-1.
14. Eyring et al. in reference: Ozonoff MB. Pediatric orthopedic radiology. W.B. Saunders Company: Philadelphia. 1992. p. 181. (Used with permission from M.B. Ozonoff; publisher's permission requested); 1965.
15. Waldt S. Hip. In: Waldt S, Woertler K, editors. Measurements and classifications in musculoskeletal radiology. Munich: Thieme; 2013. p. 10–47.
16. Beltran LS, Rosenberg ZS, Mayo JD, et al. Imaging evaluation of developmental hip dysplasia in the young adult. AJR Am J Roentgenol. 2013;200(5):1077–88.
17. Tréguier C, Chapuis M, Branger B, et al. Pubo-femoral distance: an easy sonographic screening test to avoid late diagnosis of developmental dysplasia of the hip. Eur Radiol. 2013;23(3):836–44. Epub 2012 Oct 20. https://doi.org/10.1007/s00330-012-2635-7.
18. Hubbard AM. Imaging of pediatric hip disorders. Radiol Clin North Am. 2001;39(04):721–32.
19. Kay RM, Jaki KA, Skaggs DL. The effect of femoral rotation on the projected femoral neck-shaft angle. J Pediatr Orthop. 2000;20(6):736–9. https://doi.org/10.1097/00004694-200011000-00007.
20. Green DW, Mogekwu N, Scher DM, Handler S, Chalmers P, Widmann RF. A modification of Klein's line to improve sensitivity of the anterior-posterior radiograph in slipped capital femoral epiphysis. J Pediatr Orthop. 2009;29(5):449–53.
21. Jones CE, Cooper AP, Doucette J, et al. Southwick angle measurements and SCFE slip severity classifications are affected by frog-lateral positioning. Skeletal Radiol. 2018;47(1):79–84.
22. Fayad LM, Johnson P, Fishman EK. Multidetector CT of musculoskeletal disease in the pediatric patient: principles, techniques, and clinical applications. Radiographics. 2005;25(3):603–18.
23. Albers CE, Wambeek N, Hanke MS, Schmaranzer F, Prosser GH, Yates PJ. Imaging of femoroacetabular impingement-current concepts. J Hip Preserv Surg. 2016;3(4):245–61. https://doi.org/10.1093/jhps/hnw035.
24. Yochum and Rowe. Essentials of skeletal radiology. LWW. ISBN: 0781739462.

25. Mac-Thiong JM, Labelle H, Berthonnaud E, et al. Sagittal spinopelvic balance in normal children and adolescents. Eur Spine J. 2007;16(2):227–34. https://doi.org/10.1007/s00586-005-0013-8.
26. Tannast M, Siebenrock KA, Anderson SE. Femoroacetabular impingement: radiographic diagnosis—what the radiologist should know. Am J Roentgenol. 2012;188(6):1540–52.
27. Henebry A, Gaskill T. The effect of pelvic tilt on radiographic markers of acetabular coverage. Am J Sports Med. 2013;41(11):2599–603.
28. Hamano D, Yoshida K, Higuchi C, et al. Evaluation of errors in measurements of infantile hip radiograph using digitally reconstructed radiograph from three-dimensional MRI. J Orthop. 2019;16(3):302–6. https://doi.org/10.1016/j.jor.2019.05.004.

Knee

Maria Pilar Aparisi Gómez, Paolo Simoni, and Alberto Bazzocchi

Introduction

The knee joint undergoes significant morphological and biomechanical changes during growth.

From a morphological standpoint, the secondary epiphyseal ossification centers of the femurs and the secondary epiphyseal ossification centers of the proximal tibia are pres-

M. P. Aparisi Gómez
Department of Radiology, Auckland City Hospital, Te Toka Tumai Auckland, Auckland, New Zealand

Department of Radiology, IMSKE, Valencia, Spain
e-mail: pilara@adhb.govt.nz

P. Simoni
Pediatric Imaging Department, Reine Fabiola Children's University Hospital, Université libre de Bruxelles, Brussels, Belgium

A. Bazzocchi (✉)
Diagnostic and Interventional Radiology, IRCCS Istituto Ortopedico Rizzoli, Bologna, Italy

P. Simoni, M. P. Aparisi Gómez (eds.), *Essential Measurements in Pediatric Musculoskeletal Imaging*,
https://doi.org/10.1007/978-3-031-17735-4_9

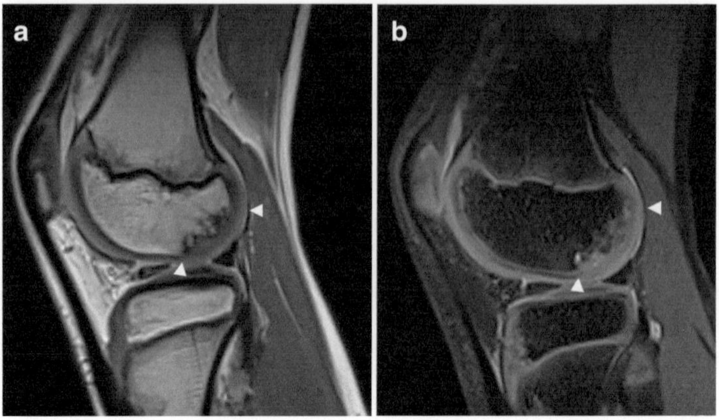

FIGURE 1 Areas of the bone marrow mimicking osteochondritis dissecans. (**a**) Sagittal T1 WI. (**b**) Sagittal PD fat sat

ent at birth [1]. The anterior apophyseal ossification center of the tibia of the anterior tuberosity occurs between 10 and 12 years of age [2], and its position may vary between different individuals which must lead to caution in interpreting measures that use it as a landmark [3]. Occasionally, the irregular maturation of the bone marrow around the secondary ossification centers bone result in many small areas of subchodral bone marrow that can mimic an osteochondritis dissecans [4] (Fig. 1a, b).

From a biomechanical perspective, growth causes a significant change in angular measurements. Therefore, the angle measurements presented in this chapter must be interpreted in an age-dependent manner. It should be noted that the measurement can be significantly affected by the degree of flexion or when performed in a standing position.

Tibiofemoral Joint

Varus–Valgus

- The tibiofemoral angle of the knee is measured on AP standing radiographs.
- Angle between two lines representing the longitudinal (anatomical) axes of the femur and tibia (Fig. 2a). The level selected to draw the longitudinal axis of the bones is midway through the diaphysis in each bone (two points can be placed in the cortices and the line drawn through the middle of them) (Fig. 2b).

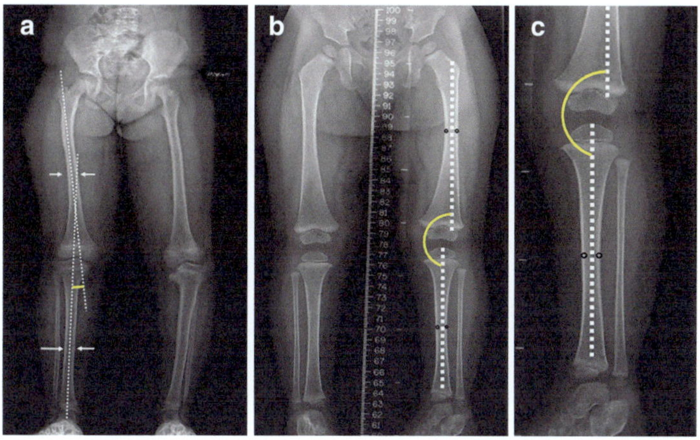

FIGURE 2 Tibiofemoral angle. (**a**) Two lines representing the longitudinal (anatomical) axes of the femur and tibia. (**b**) Points can be placed in the cortices and the line drawn through the middle of them. (**c**) Estimation if child cannot stand

Note that in children younger than 5 years, it may be difficult to obtain an AP standing radiograph (not possible in infants; in these cases, it is estimated) (Fig. 2c).

Angles are adapted to clinical settings [5]:

- From birth to 2 years: varus of 15° steadily decreasing to neutral alignment 0°.
- From 2 years to 3 years: knees move progressively from neutral alignment 0° to approximately 10 ° of valgus.
- From 3 years to 6 years: knees move progressively from 10 ° of valgus to approximately 5° of valgus (normal valgus observed in adults).

Genu valgum: tibial abduction.

Genu varum: tibial adduction.

Metadiaphyseal Angle

- The metadiaphyseal angle (MDA) [6] is used to distinguish between normal curvature of the tibia and Blount's disease (tibia vara) affecting the knee joint.
- Measured in AP standing radiographs.
- The MDA is the angle between the line joining the beaks of the metaphysis of the proximal tibia and the line perpendicular to the long axis of the tibia (drawn along the lateral aspect of the tibia) (Fig. 3a).
- An MDA $< 11°$ on radiographs in the standing position is considered normal.
- An MDA $> 11°$ is indicative of tibia vara. Please note that the appearances of the medial proximal metaphysis of the tibia should be taken into consideration for diagnosis of Blount's disease (Fig. 3b).

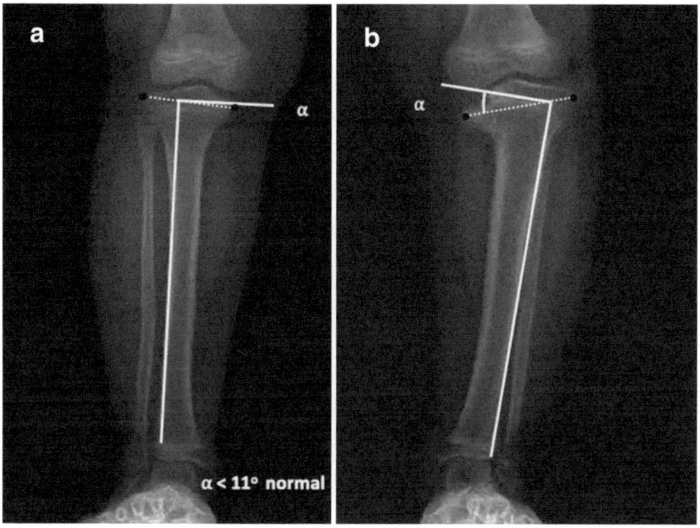

FIGURE 3 Metadiaphyseal angle. (**a**) Normal. (**b**) Tibia vara

Tibial Torsion

- Measurement taken on CT or MRI.
- Patient supine, limbs extended (not angled). Imaging is taken:
  - Below the knee—select slice just above fibular head.
  - Above the ankle—select slices including the malleoli and the fibular notch.
- Tibial torsion angle is the angle between: (Fig. 4).
  - Proximal line: line tangent to the tibial ridges.
  - Distal line: transmalleolar axis (through the center of the fibular notch).

The normal development of tibial torsion during the growth period follows a definite pattern [7]:

- At birth, there is <20° of tibial internal rotation (inward torsion of the distal tibia is considered negative).

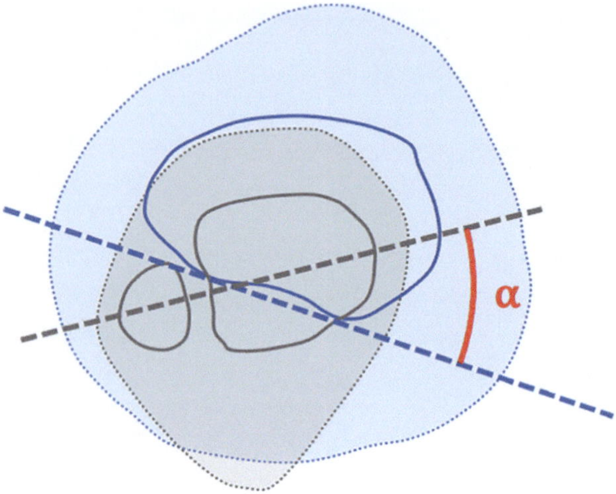

FIGURE 4 Tibial torsion angle

- From birth to 2 years of age: tibial torsion is shifted outward to 10 ° (distal tibial outward torsion is considered positive).
- From age 3 to 5 years: 27.7 SD 5.9.
- From 6 to 8 years: 32.3 SD 6.6.
- From 9 to 11 years: 33.6 SD 6.6.
- Adolescents and adults: 33.6 SD 7.3.

The physiological mean difference between measurements of the right and left sides may be 0.5 ± 2.0° (range −5° to +7°) [6].

Intercondylar Notch

- Notch index is relevant because a narrow notch is associated with ACL rupture, and a higher incidence of cyclops lesion after cruciate ligament repair.
- Measured on radiographs and MRI (coronal) (Fig. 5).
- Measurement: ratio between:
  - Width of the notch.
  - Intercondylar width.

- Normal <0.27 [8].

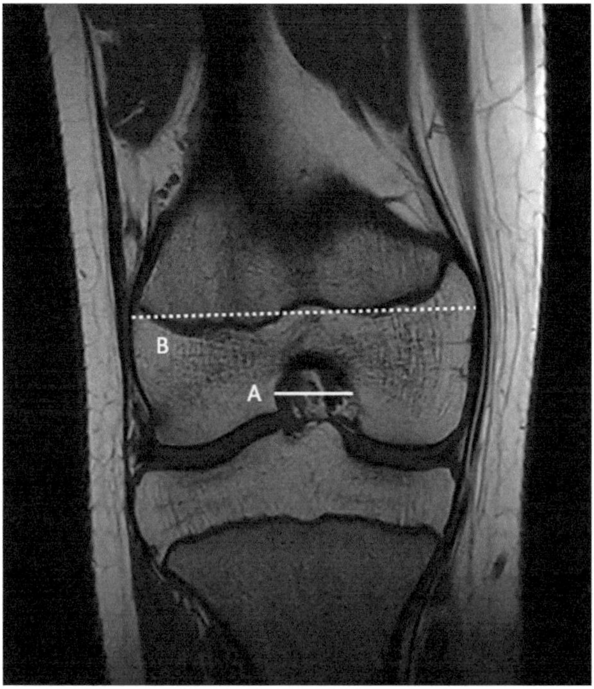

FIGURE 5 Intercondylar notch index is the ratio between *A* width of the notch, and *B* intercondylar width. A normal intercondylar notch corresponds to $A/B < 0.27$

A recent study [9] on MRI reports progressive growth of the intercondylar notch to 10 years in females and 11 on males, and stabilization at 13 years in females and 14 years in boys, with a slight reduction after this. The index showed a discrete and homogeneous reduction with age in both genders.

ACL Angles

- Younger patients have more oblique, anteriorly attached ACLs.
- Younger children tend to have partial tears and avulsion fractures of the tibial intercondylar eminence.

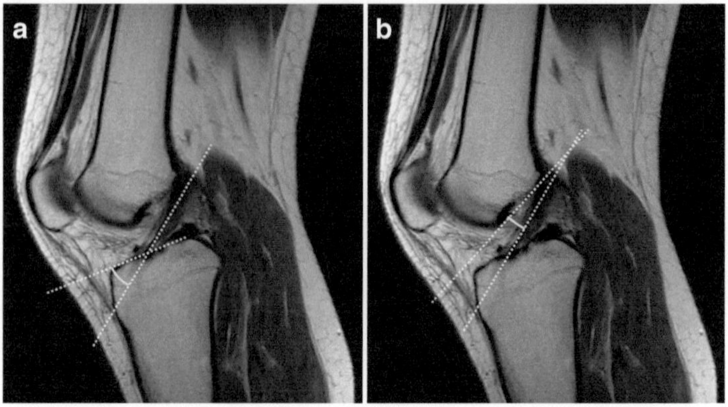

Figure 6 ACL angles. (**a**) ACL angle. (**b**) Blumensaat's angle

- Measurement of angles helps with assessment of integrity.
- ACL angle: angle between the tangent to the anterior aspect of the distal portion of the ACL and the tangent to the anterior aspect of the intercondylar eminence. Midsagittal plane (Fig. 6a).
  - Normal ~45°.
  - 44.7° ± 5.5° pediatric population [10].
- Blumensaat's angle: angle between the tangent to the anterior aspect of the distal portion of the ACL and the tangent to the intercondylar roof. Midsagittal plane (Fig. 6b).
  - Values over 10° high sensitivity and specificity for ACL tear in the pediatric population (94%/96%) [11].

PCL Angles

- Rare injury unless associated with multiple injuries. Injury patterns of the PCL in pediatric population are similar to those in adults.
- Measurements of the PCL are indirect indicators of injury to the ACL when this is not well demonstrated.

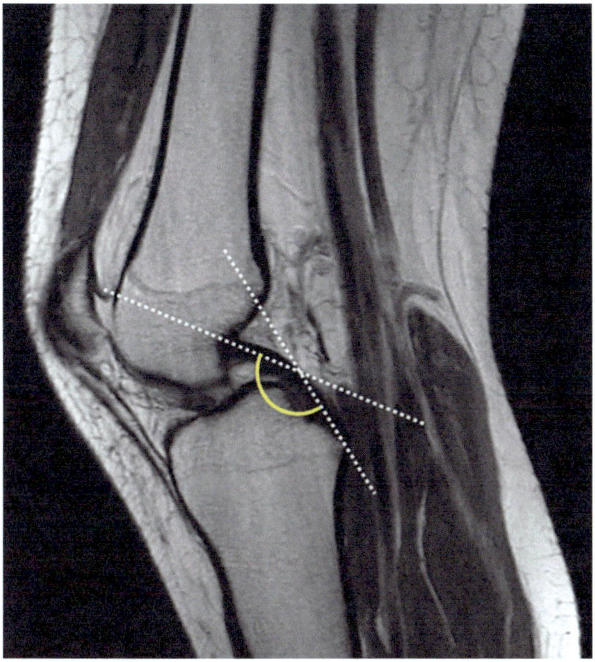

FIGURE 7 PCL angle

- PCL angle: angle between the femoral and tibial parts of the PCL (Fig. 7).
  - Normal ~123°.
  - Abnormal <106°.
- A line drawn along the tibial part of the PCL should intersect the distal femur. If this does not, the ligament is buckled and the ACL likely torn.

ACL Grafts

- A careful evaluation of skeletal age is essential to selecting the reconstruction technique. Males 15 or older and females 13 or older are candidates for transphyseal reconstruction with minimal risk of growth disturbance.

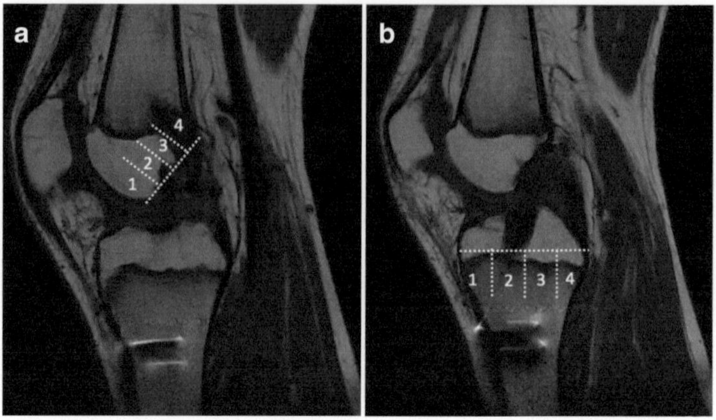

Figure 8 Tunnel positions. (**a**) Femur. (**b**) Tibia

- Younger adolescent/children should undergo physeal-sparing, partial transphyseal, and transphyseal reconstructions [12].
- Evaluation of tunnel positions (sagittal plane) [13] (Fig. 8a, b).
  - Roof of the intercondylar notch divided in four equal-length segments, numbered from anterior to posterior.
  - Lateral tibial plateau divided in four equal-length segments, numbered from anterior to posterior.
- Opening of the femoral tunnel (Fig. 9).
  - Segment 4 or posterior to it (sagittal plane).
  - Axial plane: 10 to 11 o'clock position (for the right knee) or 1 to 2 o'clock (for the left knee).
- Opening of tibial tunnel.
  - Segment 2 (sagittal plane).

If the femoral tunnel is too anterior, or the tibial tunnel too posterior, the graft will be too vertical, with instability.

If the tibial tunnel is too anterior, the graft will be too horizontal, with risk of impingement [13].

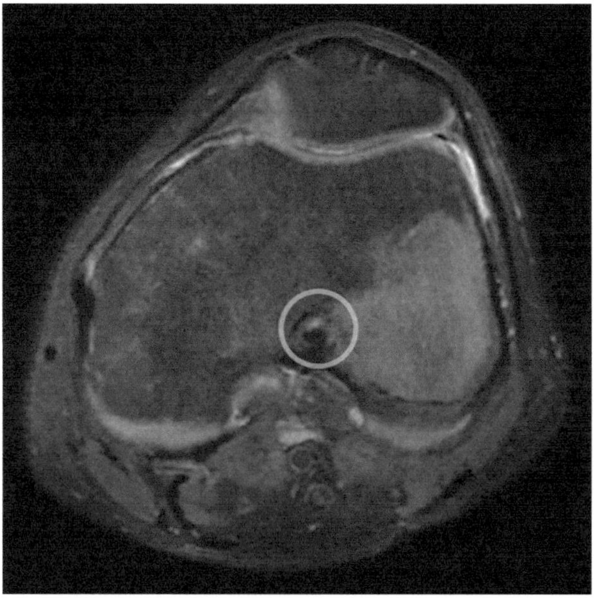

FIGURE 9 Opening of the femoral tunnel at 1 o'clock (left knee)

Discoid Meniscus

- Anatomical variant with a range of morphological features.
- US: absence of triangular configuration of meniscus, thick.
- MRI: Lateral meniscus wider than 15 mm, seen in five consecutive slices (Fig. 10).
  - Complete: Complete coverage tibial plateau. Normal attachments
  - Incomplete: Between 80 and 100% coverage plateau. Normal attachments
  - Wrisberg-type: Posterior horn thickened. The only posterior attachment of the meniscus is to the Wrisberg ligament. Hypermobile and prone to subluxation [14].

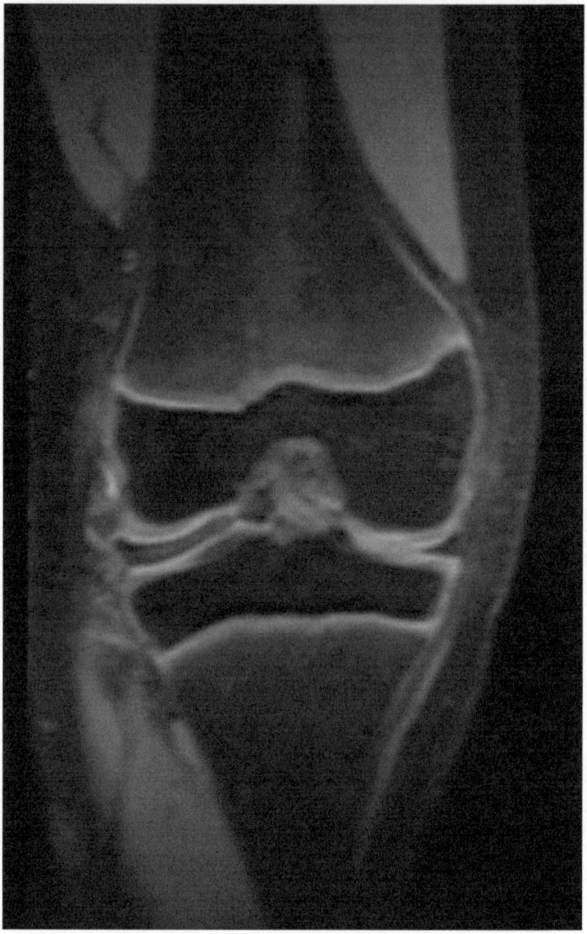

FIGURE 10 Lateral discoid meniscus

Patellofemoral Joint

Trochlear Dysplasia/Patellar Maltracking

The osseous trochlear angle increases in depth through growth; it is flatter in younger children and gains depth to assume the shape of the overlying cartilage in adolescence [15].

In a study of trochlear sulcus on MR in normal pediatric population (3–16 years), the sulcus angle measured in the cartilage surface was seen to be constant through development, and a good predictor of final trochlear shape. Final trochlear development is complete around age 8–12 [16, 17].

Cartilaginous surface is of better clinical relevance in some measurements like trochlear angle, inclination, and trochlear facet ratio [16–18] so in younger children measuring using cartilage landmarks is more representative.

Trochlear Angle (Sulcus Angle)

Radiographs

- Measurement performed in plane transverse to knee axis (sunrise view) (Fig. 11).

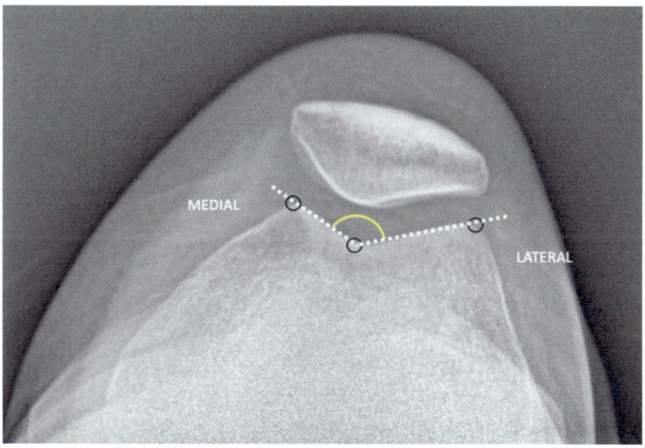

Figure 11 Trochlear angle on radiograph, sunrise view

- Angle formed by the medial and lateral articular surfaces of the trochlea.
- Lines are drawn by connecting the deepest point of the trochlea to the highest points of the medial and lateral femoral condyles.
- Range: normal up to 145°.
- Large sulcus angle (>145°) is typical of dysplasia (shallow trochlear groove) [19].

The use of these measurements on radiographs and ultrasound has been validated for adolescent populations (from 10 to 17) [20, 21].

Ultrasound

- The trochlear angle can be measured finding the equivalent cartilaginous landmarks (deepest point of cartilaginous trochlea and highest points of the cartilage at the medial and lateral femoral condyles), in the transverse plane, just below the level of the patellar apex, with the knee in 10 ° of flexion (Fig. 12a, b).
- In infants (0–24 months), the cartilaginous sulcus angle can be accurately measured with ultrasound independently of the degree of flexion of the joint [22].
- Range of normal cartilaginous angle for pediatric population (birth to 18) has been described between 134 ° and 155 ° [15, 23, 24] (Fig. 13).

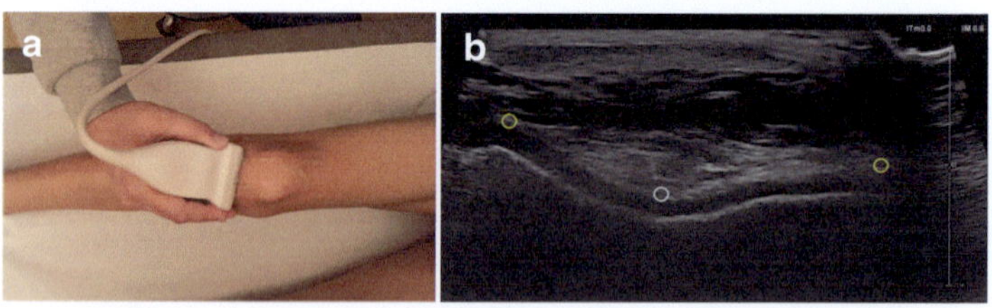

FIGURE 12 Trochlear angle on ultrasound. (**a**) Position of the transducer. (**b**) Cartilaginous landmarks: deepest point of cartilaginous trochlea (white circle) and highest points of the cartilage at the medial and lateral femoral condyles (yellow circles)

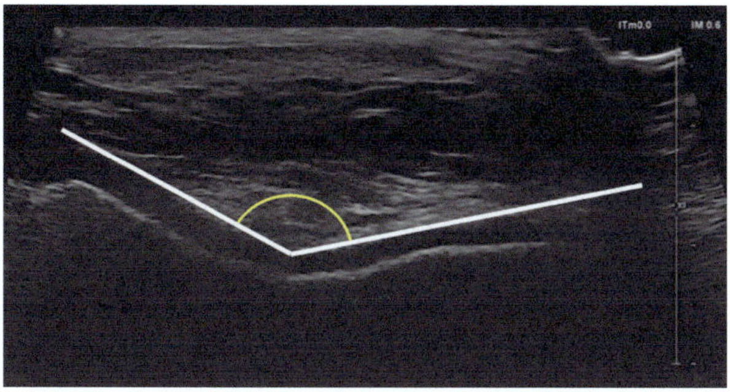

FIGURE 13 Trochlear angle measured with ultrasound

MRI

- The trochlear angle can be measured with MRI, finding the equivalent landmarks (deepest point of trochlea and highest points of the cartilage at the medial and lateral femoral condyles), in the transverse plane, with the knee in 10–20° flexion.
- Cartilaginous or osseous landmarks can be used. There is no consensus as to where to measure: generally deepest part of the trochlea or most proximal slice where trochlea is fully covered with cartilage in more mature knees (Fig. 14a).
- Cartilaginous surface is of more clinical relevance [16–18] (Fig. 14b).
- Range of normal cartilaginous angle for pediatric population (8–18 years of age) has been described as 138.2° ± 9.5.
- Range of normal osseous angle for pediatric population (8–18 years of age) has been described as 133.4° ± 12.4 [18].

Lateral Trochlear Inclination

- Measured on MRI, on the most superior axial image that includes the trochlear cartilage [25] (Fig. 15).
- Angle described by two lines:
  - Line tangent to the lateral trochlear facet surface.
  - Line tangent to the posterior surface of the femoral condyles.

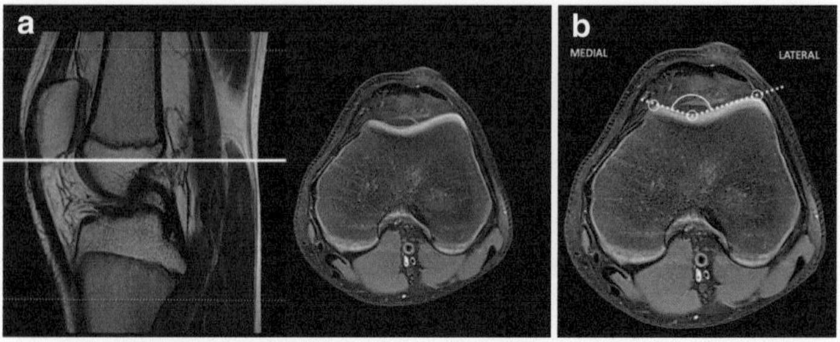

FIGURE 14 Trochlear angle. MRI assessment. (**a**) Level of measurement. (**b**) Landmarks for measurement (transverse plane)

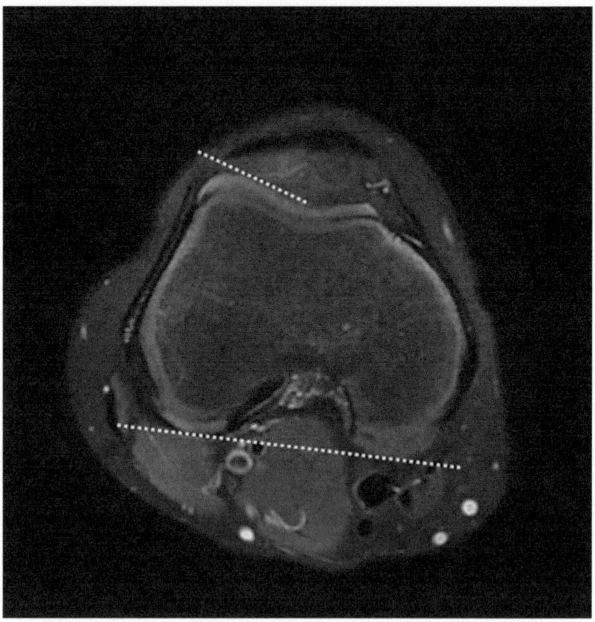

FIGURE 15 Lateral trochlear inclination

- Normal >11°.
- Abnormal <11°.

Trochlear Depth

Radiographs

- Measured 1 cm distal to the upper limit of the trochlea in true lateral projection (posterior borders of condyles overlap). Small rotations induce significant error [26] (Fig. 16).
- Distance from anterior margin of the most anterior condyle to the trochlear floor.

To fix the problem of the positioning (small rotations), the formula GM + GT/2 can be used, where GM is the distance from the trochlear floor to the anterior margin of the medial condyle and GT the distance from the trochlear floor to the anterior margin of the lateral condyle. The distances from the

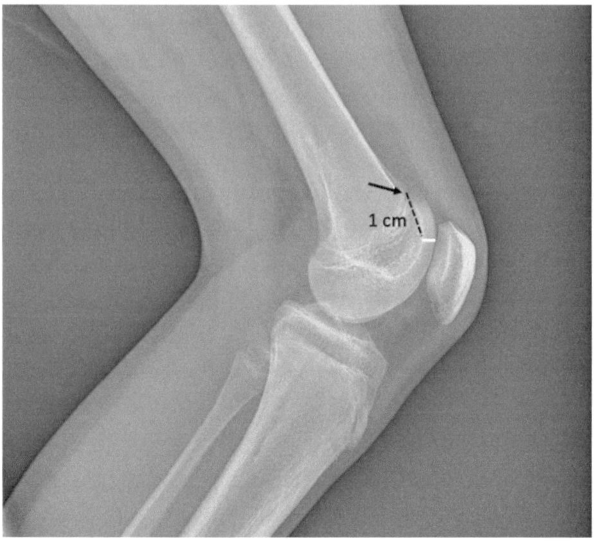

FIGURE 16 Trochlear depth on true lateral radiograph (white line). This should be measured 1 cm below the upper limit of the trochlea (black arrow - coincides with the physeal line)

trochlear floor to the anterior margin of each condyle are averaged [27].

- Normal >3 mm [28] (between 3 and 5 mm, there may be hypoplasia).
- Abnormal <3 mm.

US/CT/MRI

- Measured 3 cm above the tibiofemoral joint line.
- Use bone landmarks [29].
- Two possible ways to measure:
  - Maximum distance between a line that connects the highest points of lateral and medial facets and the deepest point of the trochlear sulcus (US, CT, and MRI).
  - Measure distances relative to and perpendicular to a line tangent to the posterior surface of the femoral condyles. The trochlear depth is calculated measuring the mean of the maximum anteroposterior distance of the lateral and medial femoral condyles (highest points from the line tangent to the posterior surface of the femoral condyles) minus the distance measured from the line tangent to the posterior surface of the femoral condyles to the deepest point of the trochlear groove (deepest point of the sulcus) (CT and MRI) (Fig. 17).
- Normal >3 mm [28] (between 3 and 5 mm, there may be hypoplasia).
- Abnormal <3 mm.

Trochlear Facet Ratio

- Measured 3 cm above the tibiofemoral joint line (RX/CT/MRI) (Fig. 18a, b).

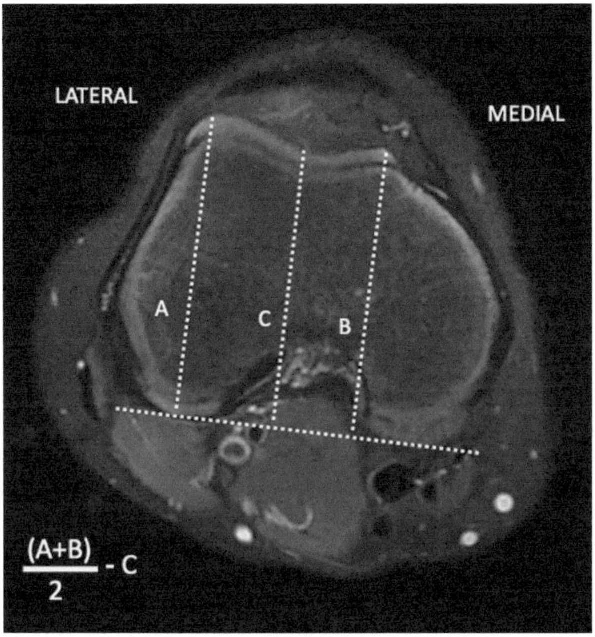

FIGURE 17 Trochlear depth on MRI, transverse plane. *A* Highest point of the lateral condyle, *B* highest point of the medial condyle, *C* deepest point of the sulcus

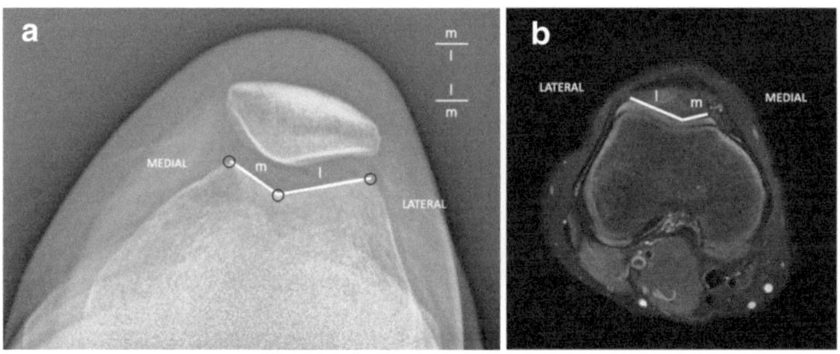

FIGURE 18 Trochlear facet ratio. (**a**) Radiograph, sunrise view. (**b**) MRI, transverse plane. *m* medial trochlear facet, *l* lateral trochlear factet

- Comparison of length of the medial and lateral facets (ratio between facet length). Ratio can be obtained:
  - Medial/lateral: abnormal ratio < 0.4 (normal >0.4).
  - Lateral/medial: abnormal ratio > 1.7 (normal <1.7) [30].

Tibial Tuberosity to Trochlear Groove Distance (TT- TG)

- Measures the position of the tibia in relation to the femoral trochlea: measures the lateral pull on the patella (if not compensated by the vastus medialis, there is risk of subluxation).
- This distance increases with age in the pediatric population [31].
- TT-TG: horizontal distance between the midpoint of the anterior aspect of the tibial tuberosity and the deepest part of the trochlear groove [20].
- Needs two superimposed sections (CT/MRI):
  - Through tibial tubercle.
  - Through deepest point of the trochlea.
- Measurement:
  - Distance from the inferior point of the patellar articular surface to a line tangent to the posterior surface of the femoral condyles.
  - Perpendicular line through tibial tubercle.
  - Perpendicular line though deepest point trochlea.

The distance between these two perpendicular lines is measured (Fig. 19).

A slight discrepancy in measurements between CT and MRI is noted, mainly due to the definition of landmarks. On MRI, the measurement can be performed using the cartilage surface in the trochlea (most proximal axial slice where trochlea is fully covered with cartilage) and the patellar tendon attachment (midpoint of the tendon in slice in which this is fully attached) – this has been labeled as "functional TT-TG" [32].

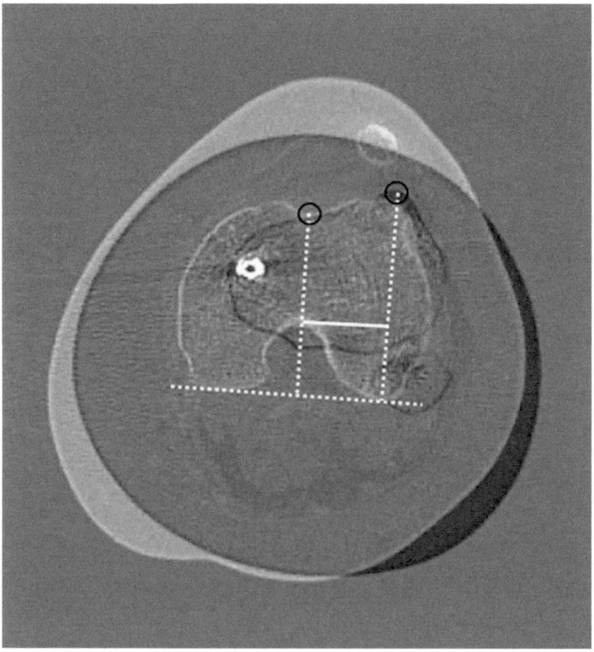

Figure 19 Tibial tuberosity to trochlear groove distance (TT-TG) (bold white line). Measured on composed CT image (superimposition of plane through the tibial tubercle and plane through deepest point of the trochlea)

- Normal <15 mm.
- Abnormal >20 mm.
- (15–20 mm borderline).

Patellar Position Assessment

Vertical Position

Koshino and Sugimoto

- Best method for children under ~13 (skeletally immature—patella not completely ossified).

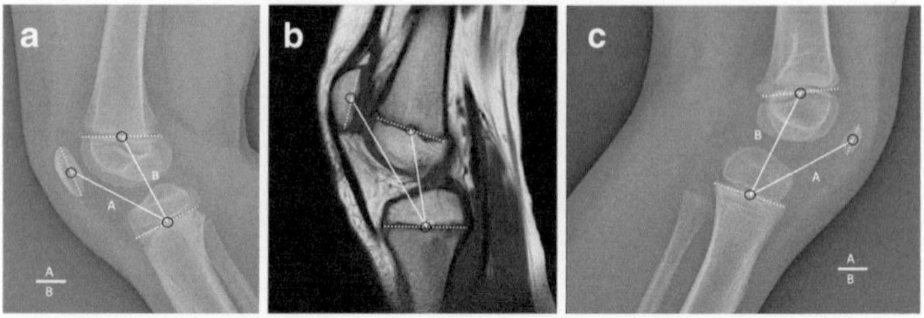

Figure 20 Assessment of vertical patellar position. Koshino and Sugimoto. (**a**) Radiograph, lateral view, 7-year-old. (**b**) MRI, sagittal plane, 12-year-old. (**c**) Radiograph, lateral view, 5-year-old. *A* distance from the midpoint of the patella to the midpoint of the proximal tibial physis, *B* distance from the midpoint of the distal femoral physis to the midpoint of the proximal tibial physis

- Performed on radiographs and MRI (Fig. 20a–c).
- The distance from the midpoint of the patella to the midpoint of the proximal tibial physis (patella-tibial) is compared from the distance from the midpoint of the distal femoral physis to the midpoint of the proximal tibial physis (femorotibial).
- Normal range patella-tibial/femorotibial ratio is 0.99–1.20 [33].

Insall-Salvati

- Useful after skeletal maturation (over ~13 years of age).
- This method can be used on MRI in younger children (using cartilage margins).
- Measurement (Fig. 21a, b):
  - Length of patellar tendon measured along the posterior edge (from patellar margin to insertion in tibial tuberosity).
  - Diagonal length of the patella.
  - Patellar tendon and patellar lengths should be nearly equal.

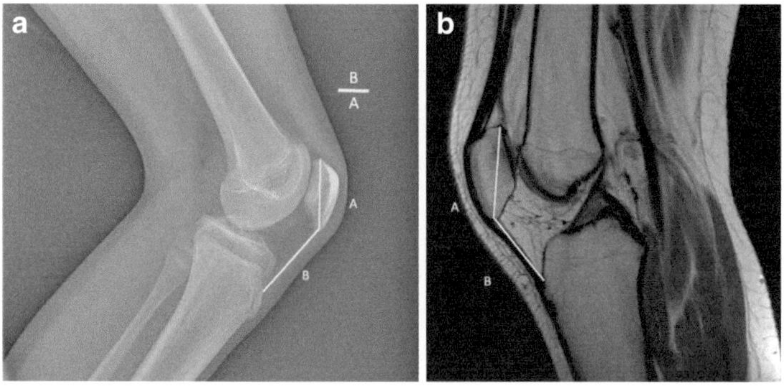

FIGURE 21 Assessment of vertical patellar position. Insall-Salvati. (**a**) Radiograph, lateral view. (**b**) MRI, sagittal plane. *A* diagonal length of the patella, *B* length of the patellar tendon

- Normal radiographic ratio range 1.02 ± 0.13.
- Patella alta ratio > 1.2 (radiographs) > 1.3 (MRI).
- Patella baja ratio < 0.8 [34, 35].

Variations of Insall-Salvati can be used in adolescents:
Caton-Deschamps

- Solves the problem in patients with a long non-articulating inferior patellar facet.
- Measurement (ratio) (Fig. 22a, b):
  - Distance from anterosuperior angle of tibia to inferior margin of the patellar articular surface.
  - Length of patellar articular surface.
- Normal 0.6–1.3.
- Patella alta >1.2.
- Patella baja <0.6 [36, 37].

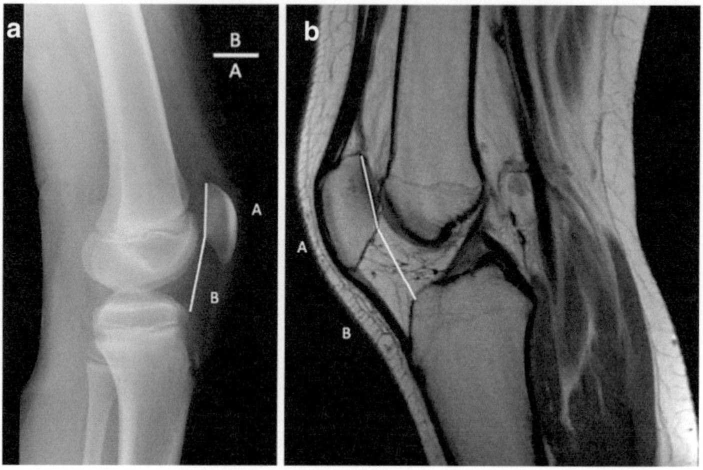

FIGURE 22 Assessment of vertical patellar position. Caton-Deschamps. (**a**) Radiograph, lateral view. (**b**) MRI, sagittal plane. *A* length of patellar articular surface, *B* distance from the anterosuperior angle of the tibia to the inferior margin of the patellar articular surface

Grelsamer-Meadows (modified Insall-Salvati)

- Diminish errors from morphological variations of the patella.
- Avoids using the anterosuperior angle of the tibia (may be absent).
- Measurement (ratio) (Fig. 23a, b):
  - Distance from inferior margin of patellar articular surface to distal insertion of patellar ligament (tibial tuberosity).
  - Length of patellar articular surface.
- Normal <2.
- Patella alta >2 [38].

Blackburne-Peel

- Measurement (ratio) (Fig. 24a, b):
  - Distance from the inferior point of the patellar articular surface to a line through the articular surface of the

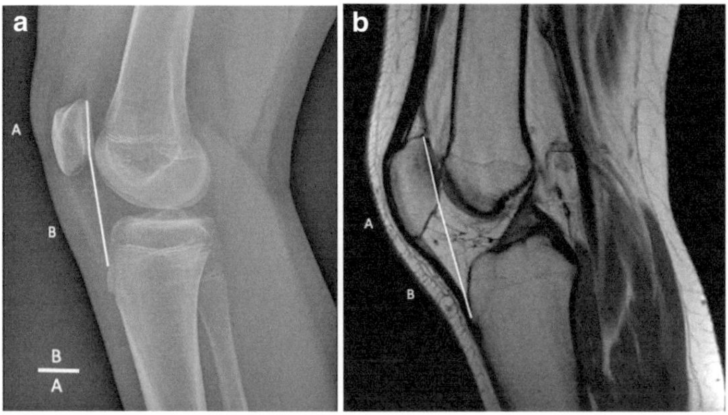

FIGURE 23 Assessment of vertical patellar position. Grelsamer-Meadows (modified Insall-Salvati). (**a**) Radiograph, lateral view. (**b**) MRI, sagittal plane. *A* length of the patellar articular surface, *B* distance from the inferior margin of the patellar articular surface to distal insertion of the patellar ligament

tibia, from the anterior and posterior margins of the medial tibial plateau.
  - Length of patellar articular surface.

- Normal 0.8–1.0.
- Patella alta >1.0.
- Patella baja <0.8 [39].

Horizontal Position

Measurements of the horizontal position and assessment of patellar maltracking in the horizontal plane have not been validated in the pediatric population. These are the congruence angle, axial linear patellar displacement, and measurements of the patellar tilt [40].

Variability is wide for adults; many of the measurements influenced in different degrees by quadriceps contraction, knee extension, and effusion [41, 42]. They are mainly used in kinematic studies.

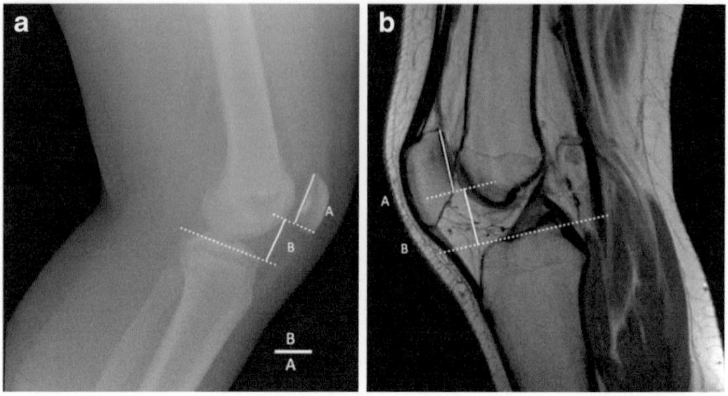

FIGURE 24 Assessment of vertical patellar position. Blackburne-Peel. (**a**) Radiograph, lateral view. (**b**) MRI, sagittal plane. *A* length of patellar articular surface, *B* distance from the inferior margin of the articular surface of the patella to a line through the articular surface of the tibia

References

1. Koifman A, Lefebvre J. Appearance of secondary ossification points and age determination of bone. Arch Fr Pediatr. 1956;13:1101–5.
2. Vergara-Amador E, Davalos Herrera D, Moreno LÁ. Radiographic features of the development of the anterior tibial tuberosity. Radiologia. 2016;58:294–300. https://doi.org/10.1016/j.rx.2016.01.005.
3. D'Amore T, Tanaka MJ, Cosgarea AJ. When and how far to move the tibial tuberosity in patients with patellar instability. Sports Med Arthrosc Rev. 2017;25:78–84. https://doi.org/10.1097/JSA.0000000000000146.
4. Laor T, Jaramillo D. MR imaging insights into skeletal maturation: what is normal? Radiology. 2009;250:28–38. https://doi.org/10.1148/radiol.2501071322.
5. Salenius P, Vankka E. The development of the tibiofemoral angle in children. J Bone Joint Surg Am. 1975;57:259–61.
6. Levine AM, Drennan JC. Physiological bowing and tibia vara. The metaphyseal-diaphyseal angle in the measurement of bowleg deformities. J Bone Joint Surg Am. 1982;64:1158–63.

7. Kristiansen LP, Gunderson RB, Steen H, Reikerås O. The normal development of tibial torsion. Skelet Radiol. 2001;30:519–22. https://doi.org/10.1007/s002560100388.
8. Botchu R, Obaid H, Rennie W. Correlation between trochlear dysplasia and the notch index. J Orthop Surg (Hong Kong). 2013;21:290–3. https://doi.org/10.1177/230949901302100305.
9. Lima FM, Debieux P, Aihara AY, et al. The development of the intercondylar notch in the pediatric population. Knee. 2020;27:747–54. https://doi.org/10.1016/j.knee.2020.04.020.
10. Reid JC, Yonke B, Tompkins M. The angle of inclination of the native ACL in the coronal and sagittal planes. Knee Surg Sports Traumatol Arthrosc. 2017;25:1101–5. https://doi.org/10.1007/s00167-017-4419-8.
11. Murao H, Morishita S, Nakajima M, Abe M. Magnetic resonance imaging of anterior cruciate ligament (ACL) tears: diagnostic value of ACL-tibial plateau angle. J Orthop Sci. 1998;3:10–7. https://doi.org/10.1007/s007760050016.
12. Perkins CA, Willimon SC. Pediatric anterior cruciate ligament reconstruction. Orthop Clin N Am. 2020;51:55–63. https://doi.org/10.1016/j.ocl.2019.08.009.
13. Wörtler K. MRT des Kniegelenks. Radiologe. 2007;47:1131–46. https://doi.org/10.1007/s00117-007-1581-x.
14. Fox MG. MR imaging of the meniscus: review, current trends, and clinical implications. Radiol Clin N Am. 2007;45:1033–53. https://doi.org/10.1016/j.rcl.2007.08.009.
15. Nietosvaara Y. The femoral sulcus in children. An ultrasonographic study. J Bone Joint Surg Br. 1994;76:807–9.
16. Richmond CG, Shea KG, Burlile JF, et al. Patellar-trochlear morphology in pediatric patients from 2 to 11 years of age: a descriptive analysis based on computed tomography scanning. J Pediatr Orthop. 2020;40:e96–e102. https://doi.org/10.1097/BPO.0000000000001405.
17. Trivellas M, Kelley B, West N, et al. Trochlear morphology development: study of normal pediatric knee MRIs. J Pediatr Orthop. 2021;41:77–82. https://doi.org/10.1097/BPO.0000000000001697.
18. Düppe K, Gustavsson N, Edmonds EW. Developmental morphology in childhood patellar instability: age-dependent differences on magnetic resonance imaging. J Pediatr Orthop. 2016;36:870–6. https://doi.org/10.1097/BPO.0000000000000556.
19. Brattstroem H. Shape of the intercondylar groove normally and in recurrent dislocation of patella. A clinical and x-ray-anatomical investigation. Acta Orthop Scand Suppl. 1964;68(SUPPL 68):1–148.

20. Dejour H, Walch G, Nove-Josserand L, Guier C. Factors of patellar instability: an anatomic radiographic study. Knee Surg, Sports Traumatol Arthrosc. 1994;2:19–26. https://doi.org/10.1007/BF01552649.
21. Fithian DC, Paxton EW, Stone ML, et al. Epidemiology and natural history of acute patellar dislocation. Am J Sports Med. 2004;32:1114–21. https://doi.org/10.1177/0363546503260788.
22. Mizobuchi RR, Galbiatti JA, Quirici Neto F, et al. Ultrasonographic study of the femoropatellar joint and its attachments in normal infants from birth to 24 months of age: part I. J Pediatr Orthop B. 2007;16:262–5. https://doi.org/10.1097/BPB.0b013e32809256d0.
23. Nietosvaara AY, Aalto KA. Ultrasonographic evaluation of patellar tracking in children. Clin Orthop Relat Res. 1993;(297):62–4.
24. Nietosvaara Y, Aalto K. The cartilaginous femoral sulcus in children with patellar dislocation: an ultrasonographic study. J Pediatr Orthop. 1997;17:50–3.
25. Carrillon Y, Abidi H, Dejour D, et al. Patellar instability: assessment on MR images by measuring the lateral trochlear inclination-initial experience. Radiology. 2000;216:582–5. https://doi.org/10.1148/radiology.216.2.r00au07582.
26. Koëter S, Bongers EMHF, de Rooij J, van Kampen A. Minimal rotation aberrations cause radiographic misdiagnosis of trochlear dysplasia. Knee Surg Sports Traumatol Arthrosc. 2006;14:713–7. https://doi.org/10.1007/s00167-005-0031-4.
27. Malghem J, Maldague B. Depth insufficiency of the proximal trochlear groove on lateral radiographs of the knee: relation to patellar dislocation. Radiology. 1989;170:507–10. https://doi.org/10.1148/radiology.170.2.2911676.
28. Ali SA, Helmer R, Terk MR. Analysis of the patellofemoral region on MRI: Association of Abnormal Trochlear Morphology with Severe Cartilage Defects. Am J Roentgenol. 2010;194:721–7. https://doi.org/10.2214/AJR.09.3008.
29. van Huyssteen AL, Hendrix MRG, Barnett AJ, et al. Cartilage-bone mismatch in the dysplastic trochlea. An MRI study. J Bone Joint Surg Br. 2006;88:688–91. https://doi.org/10.1302/0301-620X.88B5.16866.
30. Pfirrmann CW, Zanetti M, Romero J, Hodler J. Femoral trochlear dysplasia: MR findings. Radiology. 2000;216:858–64. https://doi.org/10.1148/radiology.216.3.r00se38858.
31. Dickens AJ, Morrell NT, Doering A, et al. Tibial tubercle-trochlear groove distance: defining normal in a pediatric pop-

ulation. J Bone Joint Surg Am. 2014;96:318–24. https://doi.org/10.2106/JBJS.M.00688.
32. Schoettle PB, Zanetti M, Seifert B, et al. The tibial tuberosity–trochlear groove distance; a comparative study between CT and MRI scanning. Knee. 2006;13:26–31. https://doi.org/10.1016/j.knee.2005.06.003.
33. Koshino T, Sugimoto K. New measurement of patellar height in the knees of children using the epiphyseal line midpoint. J Pediatr Orthop. 1989;9:216–8.
34. Insall J, Salvati E. Patella position in the normal knee joint. Radiology. 1971;101:101–4. https://doi.org/10.1148/101.1.101.
35. Miller TT, Staron RB, Feldman F. Patellar height on sagittal MR imaging of the knee. AJR Am J Roentgenol. 1996;167:339–41. https://doi.org/10.2214/ajr.167.2.8686598.
36. Caton J, Deschamps G, Chambat P, et al. Patella infera. Apropos of 128 cases. Rev Chir Orthop Reparatrice Appar Mot. 1982;68:317–25.
37. Thévenin-Lemoine C, Ferrand M, Courvoisier A, et al. Is the caton-deschamps index a valuable ratio to investigate patellar height in children? J Bone Joint Surg Am. 2011;93:e35. https://doi.org/10.2106/JBJS.J.00759.
38. Grelsamer RP, Meadows S. The modified insall-salvati ratio for assessment of patellar height. Clin Orthop Relat Res. 1992:170–6.
39. Blackburne JS, Peel TE. A new method of measuring patellar height. J Bone Joint Surg Br. 1977;59:241–2. https://doi.org/10.1302/0301-620X.59B2.873986.
40. Merchant AC, Mercer RL, Jacobsen RH, Cool CR. Roentgenographic analysis of patellofemoral congruence. J Bone Joint Surg Am. 1974;56:1391–6.
41. Grelsamer RP, Newton PM, Staron RB. The medial-lateral position of the patella on routine magnetic resonance imaging: when is normal not normal? Arthroscopy. 1998;14:23–8. https://doi.org/10.1016/s0749-8063(98)70116-1.
42. Meyers AB, Laor T, Sharafinski M, Zbojniewicz AM. Imaging assessment of patellar instability and its treatment in children and adolescents. Pediatr Radiol. 2016;46:618–36. https://doi.org/10.1007/s00247-015-3520-8.

Ankle and Foot

Giulia Negro, Paolo Simoni, and Hilary Umans

Introduction

Radiological evaluation of the ankle and foot provides essential information for diagnosing congenital and developmental anomalies and guiding orthopaedic treatment.

Alignment of the ankle, hindfoot, midfoot and forefoot is best assessed separately, although they are closely related anatomically and functionally.

A knowledge of the nomenclature is essential for consistent description of foot deformities.

The ankle joint consists of the distal tibia, distal fibula and talus. Inclination of the tibial plafond as seen in the coronal

G. Negro (✉)
Pediatric Imaging Department, Reine Fabiola Children's University Hospital, Université Libre de Bruxelles,
Bruxelles, Belgium

P. Simoni
Pediatric Imaging Department, Reine Fabiola Children's University Hospital, Université Libre de Bruxelles, Brussels, Belgium

H. Umans
Albert Einstein College of Medicine Bronx, New York, NY, USA

Lenox Hill Radiology Associates, PC, NYC, USA

P. Simoni, M. P. Aparisi Gómez (eds.), *Essential Measurements in Pediatric Musculoskeletal Imaging*,
https://doi.org/10.1007/978-3-031-17735-4_10

plane indicates either valgus or varus deformity of the ankle joint. Sagittal plane deformities can be characterised either by dorsiflexion or plantar flexion, which is referred to as "calcaneus" and "equinus", respectively.

The hindfoot unit consists of the talus and calcaneus; the midfoot consists of the navicular, cuboid and cuneiforms; the forefoot consists of the metatarsals and phalanges.

Hindfoot deformities are described as varus and valgus; midfoot deformities as cavus and planus; and forefoot deformities as adduction and abduction. Inversion and eversion are complex deformities involving the whole foot [1].

In adults, the anatomical axis of the foot passes through the centre of the second metatarsal head and the centre of the calcaneal tuberosity. The mechanical axis of the foot passes through the centre of the first metatarsal head and the centre of the calcaneal tuberosity. The weight-bearing platform of the foot is represented by a triangle drawn between the centre of the first metatarsal head, the centre of the fifth metatarsal head and the centre of the calcaneal tuberosity [2] (Fig. 1).

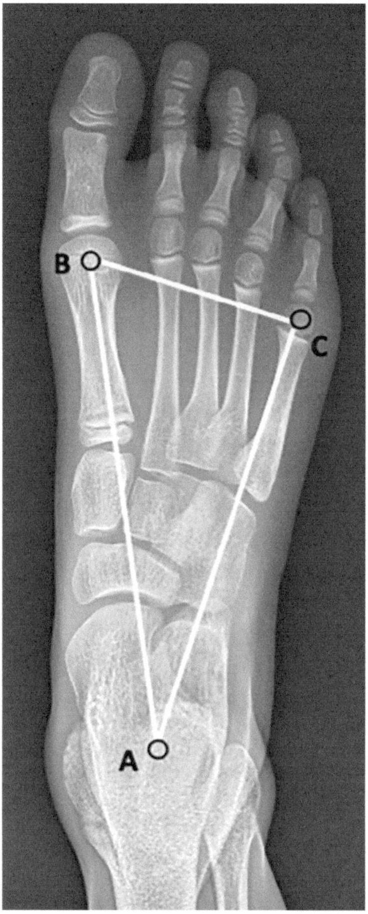

FIGURE 1 The weight-bearing platform of the foot. The weight-bearing platform of the foot is represented by a triangle drawn between the centre of the calcaneal tuberosity (*A*), the centre of the first metatarsal head (*B*) and the centre of the fifth metatarsal head (*C*)

Ankle

The ankle is a complex joint consisting of the distal tibia, distal fibula and talus, whose relationship and normal values have not been specifically validated in children.

In the anteroposterior (AP) and lateral (LAT) projections of the ankle joint, the inclination of the distal tibial articular surface can be assessed by the lateral and anterior distal tibial angles. The lateral inclination of the lateral joint surface of the distal tibia is called the "ankle valgus" (as opposed to the "ankle varus").

To assess the relationship between the distal fibula, distal tibia and talus, we can refer to some measurements traditionally used in the assessment of ankle syndesmosis injuries, such as total clear space, tibiofibular overlap, medial clear space and talocrural angle. They are performed on a mortise view, an AP projection of the ankle with the foot rotated inward 10–20° [2]. In the mortise view, the base of the fifth metatarsal bone projects vertically under the centre of the talar dome.

Lateral Distal Tibial Angle

(Fig. 2)

- Lines: distal tibial articular surface/long axis of the tibia.
- In the AP view: in young children, there is usually a slight valgus angle that approaches 90° by age 10; 89° ± 3° in adulthood [1, 3].

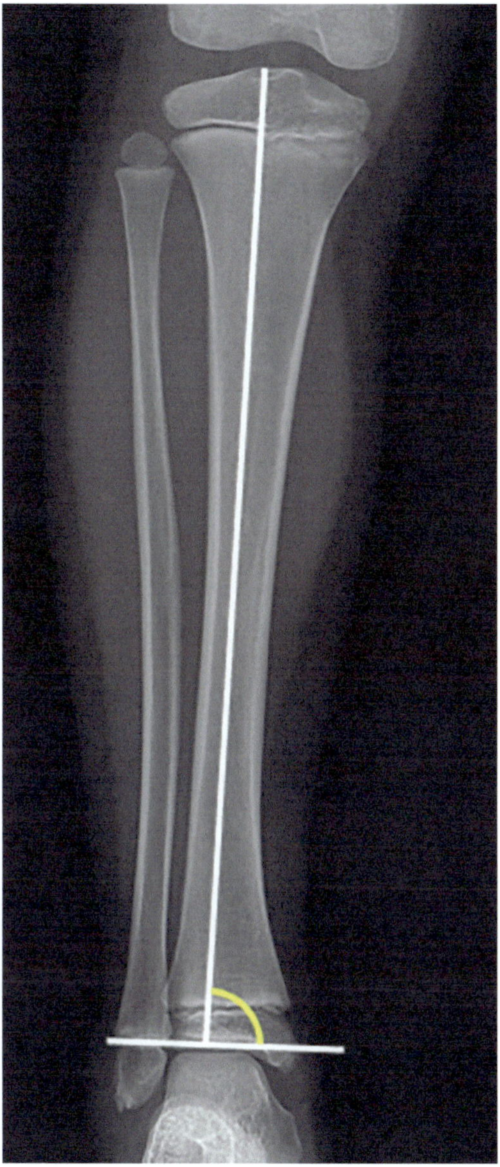

FIGURE 2 Lateral distal tibial angle. The angle between the lines drawn with respect to the distal tibial articular surface and the long axis of the tibia, in the AP view

Anterior Distal Tibial Angle

(Fig. 3)

- Lines: distal tibial articular surface/long axis of the tibia.
- In the lateral view: 79.8 ± 1.60° in adulthood [4].

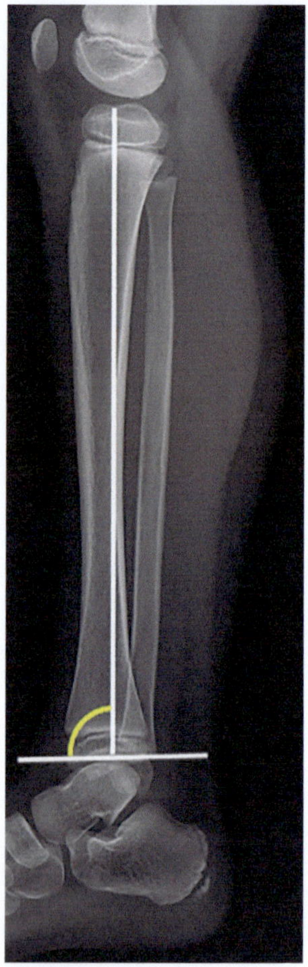

FIGURE 3 Anterior distal tibial angle. The angle between the lines drawn with respect to the distal tibial articular surface and the long axis of the tibia, in the lateral view

Total Clear Space

(Fig. 4)

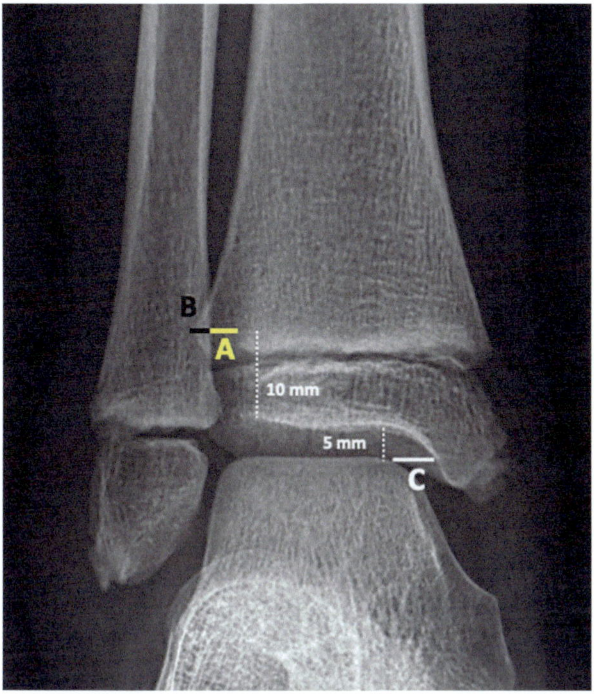

FIGURE 4 Measurement of total clear space (TCS), tibiofibular overlap (TFO) and medial clear space (MCS), in the mortise view. TCS (*A*, yellow line): distance between the medial margin of the fibular groove (posterior border of the tibia) and the medial border of the fibula, measured 10 mm (dotted line) above the tibial plafond. TFO (*B*, black line): distance between the lateral border of the distal tibia and the medial border of the fibula, measured 10 mm (dotted line) above the tibial plafond. MCS (*C*, white line): distance between the lateral border of the medial malleolus and the medial border of the talus, measured 5 mm (dotted line) below the tibial plafond

- Distance between the medial margin of the fibular groove (posterior border of the tibia) and the medial border of the fibula, measured 10 mm above the tibial plafond.
- On the mortise view: <4 mm.
- Excessive distance suggests syndesmotic injury.

Tibiofibular Overlap

- Distance between the lateral border of the distal tibia and the medial border of the fibula, measured 10 mm above the tibial plafond.
- On the mortise view: >1 mm.
- Reduced tibiofibular overlap on the mortise view suggests syndesmotic injury.

Medial Clear Space

- Distance between the lateral border of the medial malleolus and the medial border of the talus, measured 5 mm below the tibial plafond.
- On the mortise view: ≤5 mm.
- Widening of the distance suggests syndesmotic injury.

Talocrural Angle

(Fig. 5)

- Formed by a line perpendicular to the distal tibial articular surface and a line connecting the distal ends of the malleoli.
- On the mortise view: 83° ± 4°.
- Increased angle (>87°) suggests syndesmotic injury.

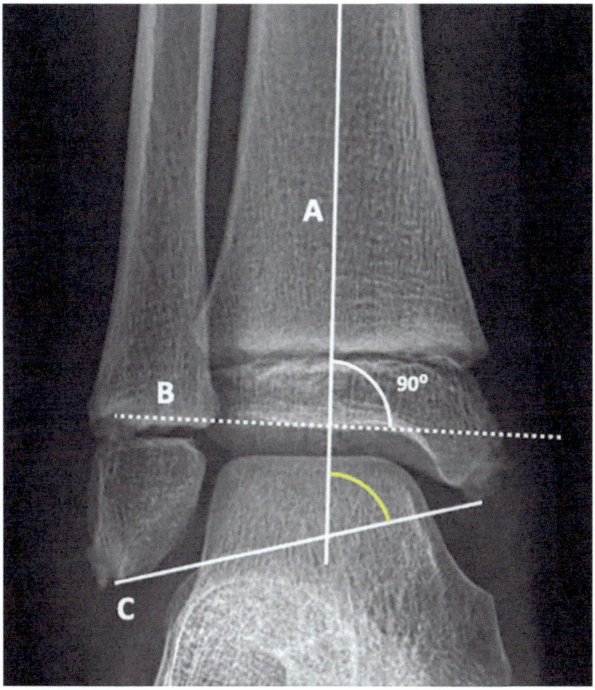

FIGURE 5 Talocrural angle. The angle formed by a line (*A*) perpendicular to the distal tibial articular surface (*B*) and a line (*C*) connecting the distal ends of the malleoli, in the mortise view

Foot

Most qualitative and quantitative assessments are based on the dorsoplantar (AP) and lateral (LAT) radiographic views, which must be obtained either in weight-bearing or simulated

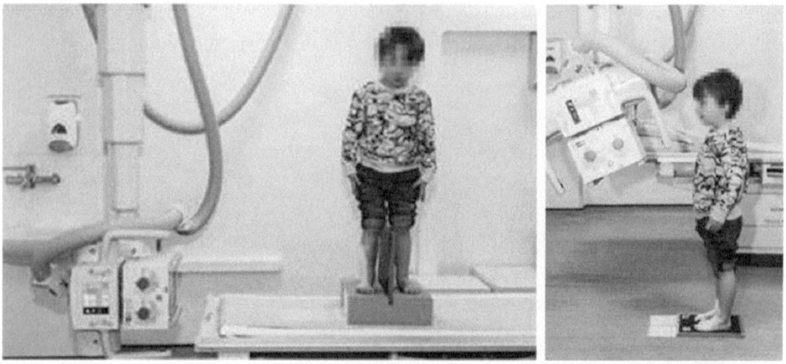

FIGURE 6 Position for lateral and AP standing radiograph. (Courtesy of Cassar-Pullicino and Davies [5])

weight-bearing (dorsiflexion stress), which allows proper configuration of the bony skeleton in its physiologic function to transmit load, adapt to surface conditions or act as a lever for progression.

The AP view is obtained with the patient standing (or in dorsiflexion stress), with the tibia perpendicular to the cassette and the central ray inclined 15° from the vertical line. The lateral view is taken with the patient standing (or in dorsiflexion stress) with the tibia parallel to the cassette (Fig. 6).

In some cases (e.g. diagnosis of foot deformities in infants, including congenital vertical talus and equinovarus), a lateral view in maximum dorsiflexion can be performed. Evaluation of the Bohler and Gissane angles requires superimposition of both malleoli, with the central beam overlying the malleoli [5].

To evaluate the coronal hindfoot alignment with the Meary and Djian methods, a Meary-Tomeno view is needed (Fig. 7): this is an anterior view of the ankle in slight medial rotation, with the heel elevated by a radiolucent wedge (2–3 cm) and the hindfoot enclosed (lead wires on the coronal plane around the malleoli) to reveal plantar support. The tibiotalar line must be horizontal. It allows a quantification of hindfoot valgus or varus and to assess non-operative corrective intervention (adding a heel pad to reduce the deformity) [6, 7]. The Saltzman and El-Khoury distance and the Lamm

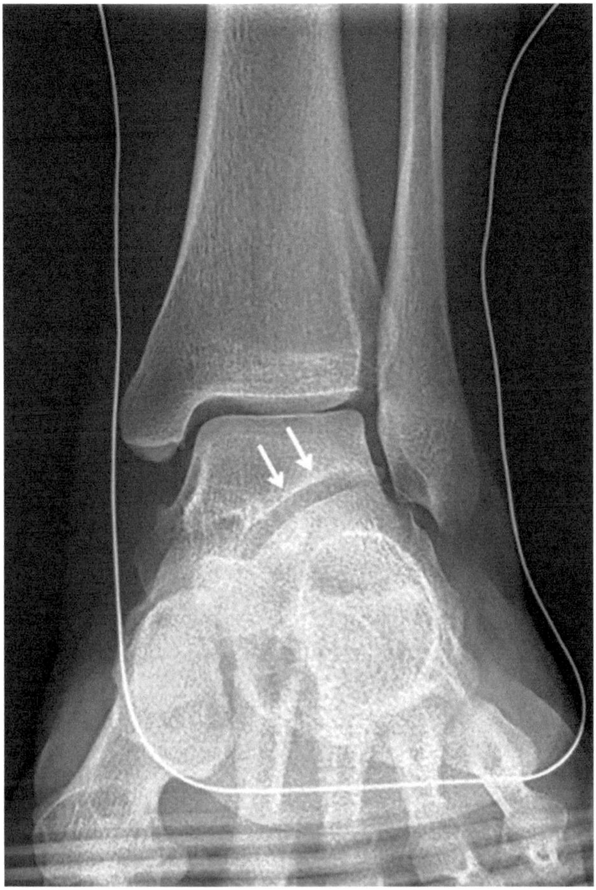

FIGURE 7 Maery-Tomeno view. The Maery-Tomeno view is an anterior view of the ankle in slight medial rotation, with the heel elevated by a radiolucent wedge and the hindfoot enclosed (lead wires perpendicular to the malleoli) to reveal plantar support. The tibiotalar line must be horizontal. Note the normal inclination (around 23°) of the subtalar joint line to the horizontal (white arrows)

angle can complete the evaluation of hindfoot deformity in a coronal view, as described below in the specific sections [8, 9]. One must be aware that the measurements taken in these views are not validated in children.

Hindfoot

Since the talus is the only bone with no direct muscular connection to the foot, its hindfoot alignment is assessed by analysing the relationship between the talus and calcaneus through the midtalar line and the midcalcaneal line.

The navicular should typically align with the talus. Malalignment of the hindfoot often results in talonavicular subluxation.

The position of the usually dorsally flexed calcaneus is described in relation to the tibia and talus by the tibiocalcaneal angle and the talocalcaneal angle, respectively. The position of the calcaneus in relation to the ground is described by both the talo-horizontal angle and the calcaneal-horizontal angle.

Hindfoot deformity in the coronal plane can be evaluated with the Meary and Djian methods [6, 7], the Saltzman and El-Khoury distance and the Lamm angle [8, 9]. These measurements, however, are not specifically validated in children.

In addition, two angles related to the morphology of the calcaneus can be used in the evaluation of calcaneal fractures: the Bohler angle and the Gissane angle.

Midtalar Line

(Fig. 8)

- In AP and lateral views, it is drawn along the central axis of the bone.
- In the AP view, it runs drawn between the midpoints of two lines through opposite points on the talus margins at the widest and narrowest points of the talus head and neck.
- In the AP view, in very young children, it runs parallel to the medial cortex of the ossification centre.
- In the AP view, in normal individuals, it passes through or slightly medial to the base of the first metatarsal.

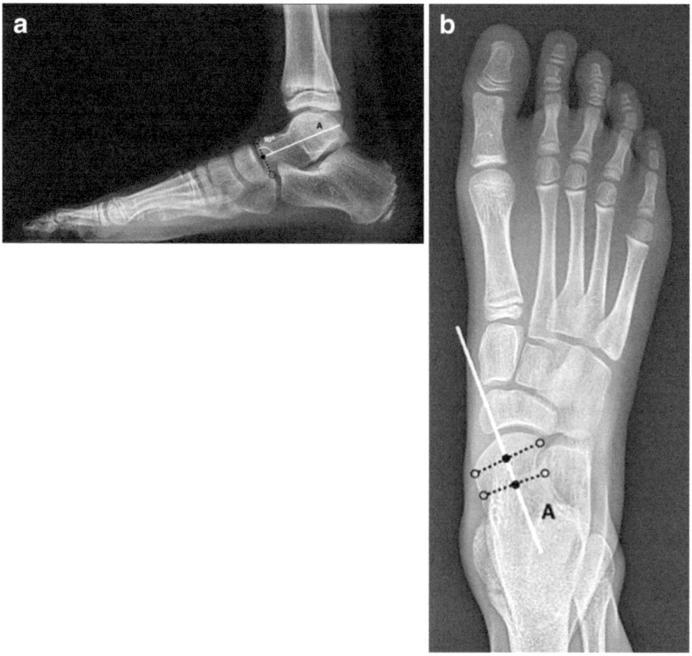

FIGURE 8 Midtalar line. (**a**) In this lateral view, the midtalar line (*A*) has been drawn as a perpendicular line through the midpoint (solid dot) of a line (dotted line) through the superior and inferior borders (circles) of the talonavicular articular surface. (**b**) In this AP view, the midtalar line (*A*) has been drawn between the midpoints (solid dots) of two lines (dotted lines) through opposite points on the talus margins at the widest and narrowest points (circles) of the talus head and neck. It passes slightly medial to the base of the first metatarsal bone

- In the hindfoot valgus, the midtalar line runs medial to the base of the first metatarsal (e.g. pes planus); in the hindfoot varus, the line runs lateral to the base of the first metatarsal (e.g. congenital equinovarus) [1].
- In the lateral view, it is drawn as a perpendicular line through the midpoint of a line through the superior and inferior borders of the talonavicular articular surface.

Midcalcaneal Line

(Fig. 9)

- In the AP and lateral views, it is drawn along the central axis of the bone.
- In the AP view, it may be drawn between the anteromedial corner of the calcaneus and the midpoint of the posterior margin of the calcaneus, or as a tangent to the lateral calcaneal cortex.
- In the AP view, in very young children, it runs parallel to the lateral cortex of the ossification centre.

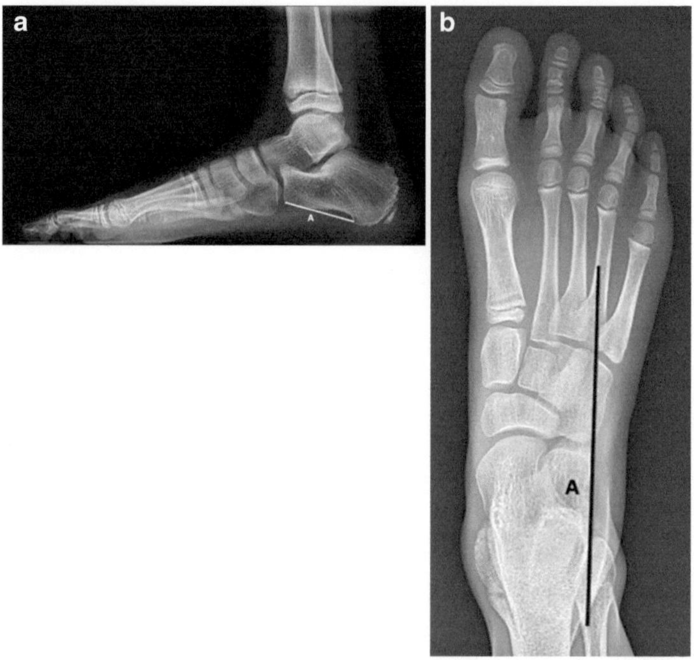

FIGURE 9 Midcalcaneal line. (**a**) In this lateral view, the midcalcaneal line (*A*) has been drawn between the anterior extension of the calcaneal tuberosity on the plantar side and the anteroinferior corner of the calcaneus that articulates with the cuboid. (**b**) In this AP view, the midcalcaneal line (*A*) has been drawn as a tangent to the lateral calcaneal cortex. It passes through the base of the fourth metatarsal

- In the AP view, in normal individuals, it passes through the base of the fourth metatarsal.
- In the lateral view, it is drawn between the anterior extension of the calcaneal tuberosity on the plantar side and the anteroinferior corner of the calcaneus that articulates with the cuboid.

Lateral Tibiocalcaneal Angle

(Fig. 10, Tables 1 and 2)

- Lines: distal tibial shaft/midcalcaneal line.
- In the lateral view: 78° (59°; 96°) in the newborn and 68° (56°; 80°) by age 4 years [10].
- In the lateral/maximum dorsiflexion view: 41° (25°; 60°) in the newborn and 52° (30°; 74°) by age 4 years [10].
- An excessive tibiocalcaneal angle is observed in equinus deformity (congenital equinovarus, rocker bottom deformity).
- A reduced tibiocalcaneal angle is observed in calcaneus deformity (calcaneocavus).

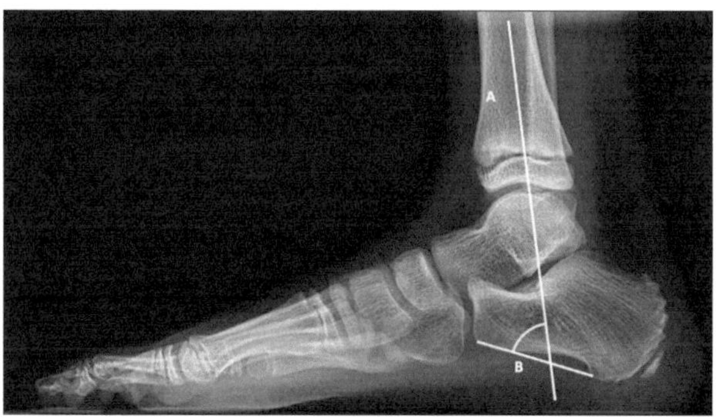

FIGURE 10 Lateral Tibiocalcaneal angle. The angle between the distal tibial shaft (*A*) and the midcalcaneal line (*B*), in the lateral view

Table 1 Changes in lateral weight-bearing tibiocalcaneal angle during growth (adapted from Vanderwilde et al. [10])

Age (years)	Mean (°)	−2SD (°)	+2SD (°)
0	77.9	59.2	96.1
1	74.3	57.9	91.2
2	71.7	56.4	87.3
3	69.5	56.3	83.5
4	67.7	56.3	80.1
5	66.8	57.1	77.8
6	66.6	58.1	76.5
7	67.1	59.7	75.1
8	67.9	61.7	74.1
9	69.3	64.7	74.1

SD standard deviation

Table 2 Changes in lateral maximum dorsiflexion tibiocalcaneal angle during growth (adapted from Vanderwilde et al. [10])

Age (years)	Mean (°)	−2SD (°)	+2SD (°)
0	41.3	24.8	59.8
1	45.4	25.7	65.9
2	48.0	27.6	69.2
3	49.7	28.9	72.3
4	51.7	30.3	73.6
5	52.6	32.6	73.4
6	52.8	34.6	71.9
7	52.2	36.2	70.4

SD standard deviation

Talocalcaneal Angle

(Fig. 11, Tables 3, 4, and 5)

- Lines: midcalcaneal/midtalar lines.
- In the AP view: 42° (27°–56°) in the newborn and 34° (24°–44°) by age 4 years [10].
- In the lateral view: 39° (23°; 56°) in the newborn, 45° (33°–57°) by age 4 years and then decreasing [10].
- In the lateral/maximum dorsiflexion view: 46° (35°–56°) in the newborn and 43 (33°–53°) by age 4 years [10].
- An excessive talocalcaneal angle (usually >45° [1]) is observed in valgus deformity (pes planus, skew foot).

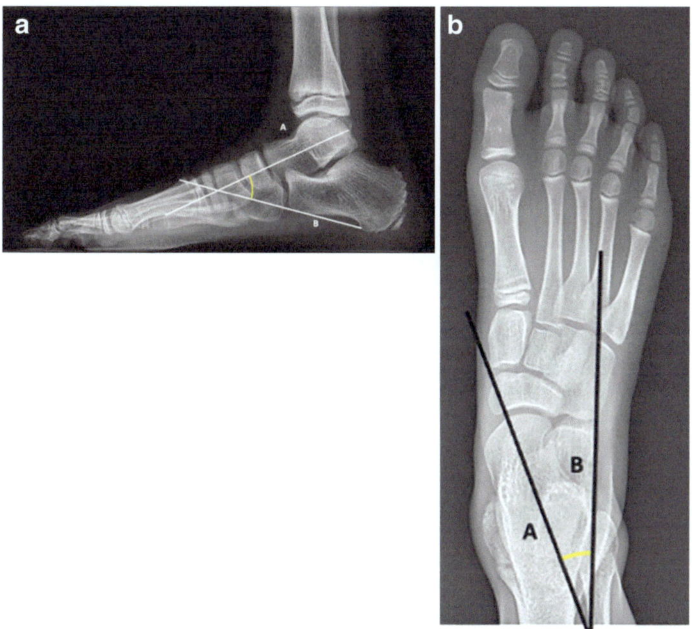

FIGURE 11 Talocalcaneal angle. (**a**) The angle between the midtalar line (*A*) and the midcalcaneal line (*B*), in the lateral view. (**b**) The angle between the midtalar line (*A*) and the midcalcaneal line (*B*), in the AP view

TABLE 3 Changes in AP weight-bearing talocalcaneal angle during growth (adapted from Vanderwilde et al. [10])

Age (years)	Mean (°)	−2SD (°)	+2SD (°)
0	41.9	27.4	56.4
1	40.1	27.1	52.9
2	37.7	26.0	49.9
3	35.7	25.4	46.8
4	33.6	24.0	44.2
5	31.7	22.2	41.3
6	29.5	19.5	39.6
7	27.1	17.5	37.0
8	24.7	14.8	35.3
9	21.6	11.2	33.4

SD standard deviation

TABLE 4 Changes in lateral weight-bearing talocalcaneal angle during growth (adapted from Vanderwilde et al. [10])

Age (years)	Mean (°)	−2SD (°)	+2SD (°)
0	38.8	23.0	55.5
1	41.2	27.1	55.5
2	43.3	29.6	56.4
3	44.4	31.6	56.9
4	45.0	32.9	56.7
5	45.3	33.5	56.1
6	44.4	33.5	55.6
7	43.7	32.5	54.8
8	42.1	30.5	53.6
9	39.7	28.4	51.4

SD standard deviation

TABLE 5 Changes in lateral maximum dorsiflexion talocalcaneal angle during growth (adapted from Vanderwilde et al. [10])

Age (years)	Mean (°)	−2SD (°)	+2SD (°)
0	45.7	34.5	56.2
1	44.8	33.8	55.0
2	43.7	33.5	54.1
3	43.0	32.9	53.4
4	42.5	32.6	52.7
5	42.1	32.1	52.0
6	41.3	31.7	51.8
7	41.4	31.0	51.9
8	40.8	30.7	51.4
9	40.3	30.4	51.4

SD standard deviation

- A reduced talocalcaneal angle (usually <20° [11]) is observed in varus deformity (congenital equinovarus, cavovarus).
- The talocalcaneal angle on lateral/maximum dorsiflexion view is a technical measure of outcome following correction of congenital equinovarus in infants who have not started to walk [5].

Talo-Horizontal Angle

(Fig. 12, Table 6)
- Lines: midtalar line/ground line.
- In the lateral view: 35° (14°–56°) in the newborn and 30° (20°–39°) by age 4 years [10].
- This measure is not used in clinical routine [5].
- An excessive talo-horizontal angle is observed in pes planus (planovalgus [2], vertical talus [5]).
- A reduced talo-horizontal angle is observed in pes cavus [2] and congenital equinovarus [5].

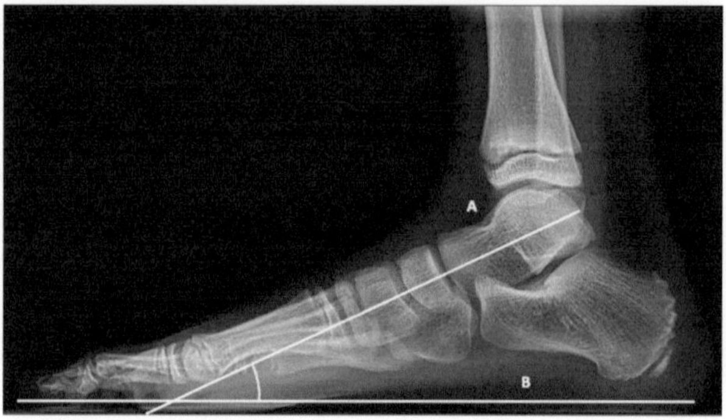

FIGURE 12 Talo-horizontal angle. The angle between the midtalar line (*A*) and the ground line (*B*), in the lateral view

TABLE 6 Changes in lateral weight-bearing talo-horizontal angle during growth (adapted from Vanderwilde et al. [10])

Age (years)	Mean (°)	−2SD (°)	+2SD (°)
0	35.1	13.5	55.7
1	33.0	15.7	49.9
2	32.1	17.9	46.1
3	31.1	19.4	42.6
4	30.0	19.7	39.1
5	28.9	19.9	37.6
6	28.1	19.4	36.4
7	26.9	17.2	35.6
8	26.1	15.7	35.6
9	25.3	13.9	36.0

SD standard deviation

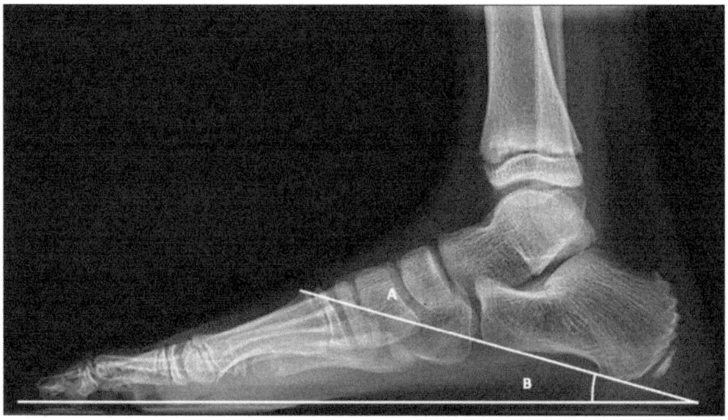

FIGURE 13 Calcaneal-horizontal angle. The angle between the midcalcaneal line (*A*) and the ground line (*B*), in the lateral view

Calcaneal-Horizontal Angle

(Fig. 13)

- Lines: midcalcaneal/ground line.
- In the lateral view: between 20° and 30° [5].
- An excessive angle (greater than 30°) is observed in congenital equinovarus, with cavus deformity, and calcaneocavus [5].
- A reduced angle (smaller than 20°) is observed in pes planovalgus [5].

Meary Method

(Fig. 14)

- In the Meary-Tomeno view.
- This method examines the projection of the tibial axis in relation to the heel contact area (divided in three portions). The tibial axis is defined by the vertical line passing through the centre of the talar dome or by the perpendicular to the tangent to the talar dome passing through the centre of the dome [6, 7].

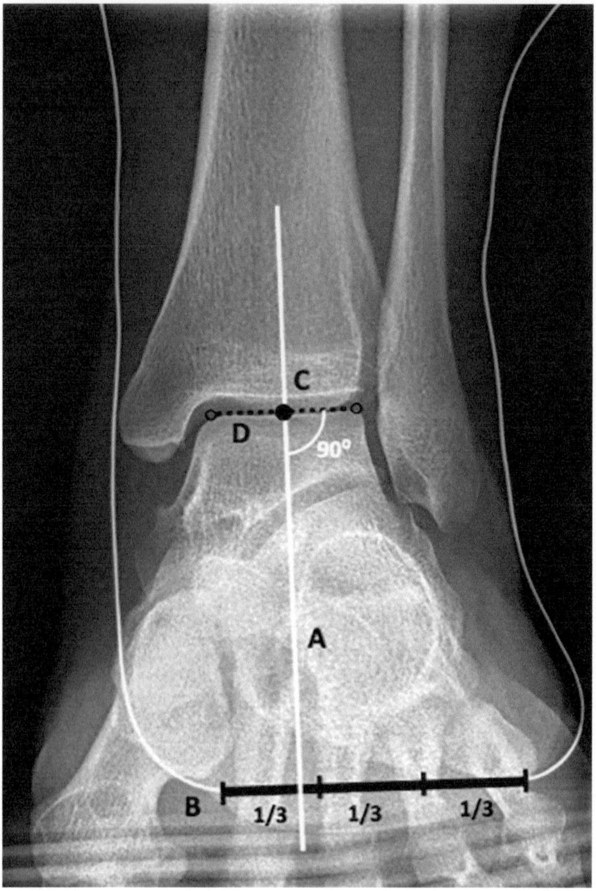

FIGURE 14 Meary method. This method examines the projection of the tibial axis (*A*) in relation to the heel contact area (*B*, divided in three portions). The tibial axis is defined in this picture by the perpendicular (*A*) to the tangent to the talar dome (*D*) passing through the centre of the dome (black dot, *C*). In normal individuals, the tibial axis intersects the heel support zone at the junction of the medial 1/3 and central 1/3. In this picture, the tibial axis intersects the heel support zone in the medial 1/3 portion (valgus of the hindfoot)

- Normal: the tibial axis intersects the heel support zone at the junction of the medial 1/3 and central 1/3; therefore, there is physiological valgus of the hindfoot.
- Valgus of the hindfoot: the tibial axis intersects the heel support zone in the medial 1/3 portion.
- Varus of the hindfoot: the tibial axis approaches the middle of the support area.

Djian Method

(Fig. 15)
- In the Meary-Tomeno view.
- The angle between the vertical and the straight line connecting the centre of the malalignment zone (subtalar joint or, more rarely, the dome of the talus) with the centre of the heel support zone is measured [7].
- Normal: physiological valgus of 3–5°.
- Valgus: Djian angle is increased.
- Varus: the Djian angle is decreased.

Saltzman and El-Khoury Distance

- The hindfoot alignment view (Fig. 16): subjects stand on a radiolucent platform with equal weight on both feet. Two positions are possible: the straight position and the natural position. In the straight position, subjects stand on the platform facing the film with the medial edge of the feet parallel and the knees extended. In the natural position, subjects stand on the platform with the imaged side in the same orientation as in the straight position and with the non-imaged side in a natural external rotation. The X-ray cassette is at an angle of 20° to the vertical. A 3×2×60 mm lead strip is placed tangential to the most posterior aspect of the heel and is oriented perpendicular to the long axis

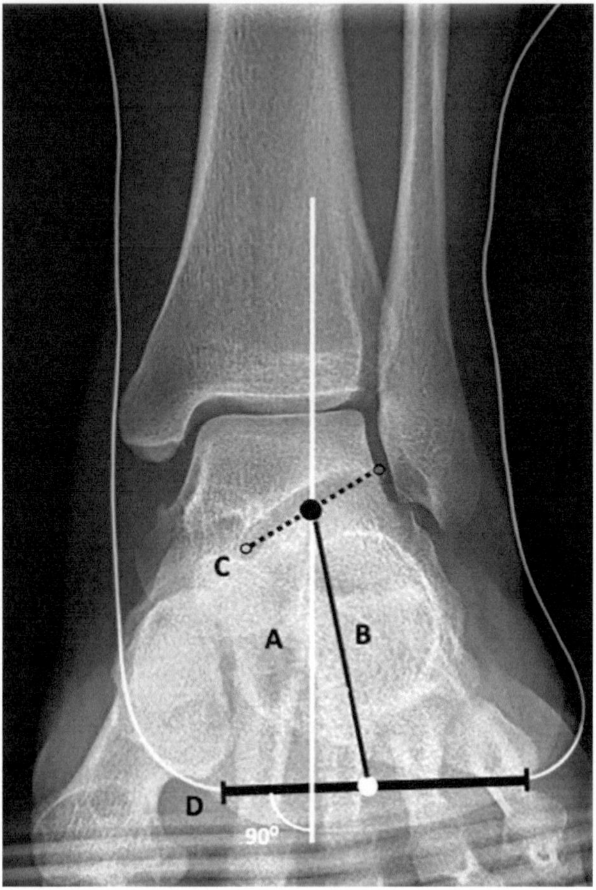

FIGURE 15 Djian method. The angle between the vertical (*A*) and the straight line (*B*) connecting the centre (black dot) of the malalignment zone (subtalar joint in this picture, line *C*) with the centre (white dot) of the heel support zone (*D*) is measured

of the foot. The X-ray tube is angled 20° from horizontal so that it is perpendicular to the film plane. The beam is centred at the level of the ankle; the field of view extends from

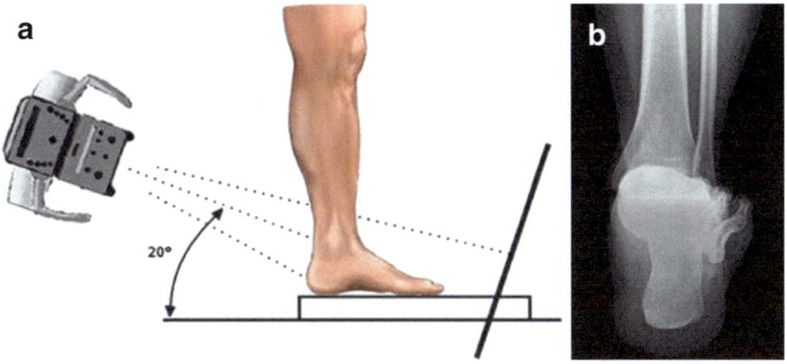

FIGURE 16 The hindfoot alignment view. (Courtesy of Reilingh et al. [12]). (**a**) Subjects stand on a radiolucent platform in the straight position or in the natural position. The X-ray cassette is at an angle of 20° to the vertical. A lead strip is placed tangential to the most posterior aspect of the heel (not pictured). The X-ray tube is angled 20° from horizontal so that it is perpendicular to the film plane. The beam is centred at the level of the ankle [8]. (**b**) Radiograph showing the hindfoot alignment view

the middle of the tibia to below the calcaneus. The distance between the source and the film is 1.016 m [8].

- The tibiocalcaneal alignment in the coronal plane (or apparent moment arm) is defined by measuring the horizontal distance on the marker line (i.e. the plane of the floor in the coronal plane) between two lines defined as follows [8]:
  - The first line is a line corresponding to the weight-bearing axis of the leg represented by the mid-longitudinal axis of the tibia (defined by bisecting the tibia 10 and 15 cm above the medial tibial plafond).
  - The second line is the perpendicular to the lead marker line passing through the lowest aspect of the calcaneus (the point under the calcaneus closest to the lead marker line).

- Apparent moment arm values are given:
  - A positive sign when the weight-bearing axis of the leg falls medial to the lowermost point of the calcaneus (valgus calcaneus).
  - A negative sign when the weight-bearing axis of the leg falls lateral to the lowermost point of the calcaneus (varus calcaneus).
- Normal values in straight position: −3.2 ± 7.2 mm [8].
- Normal values in natural position: −1.6 ± 7.2 mm [8].
- It is not validated in children.

Lamm Angle

- The long axial view (Fig. 17): the long leg calcaneal axial view captures the distal third of the tibia, the subtalar joint and the calcaneus. In this view, the patient is in the ski-

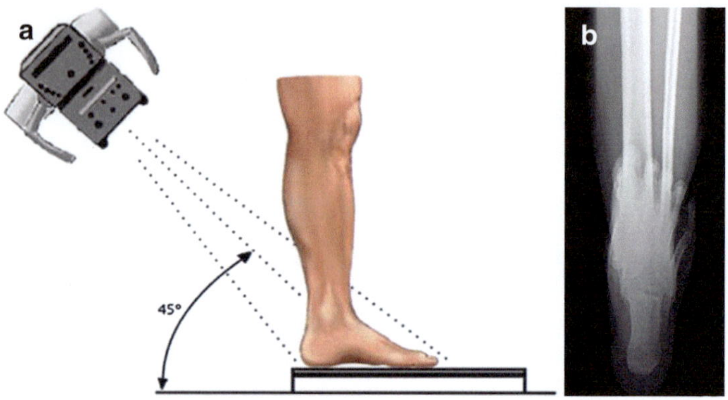

FIGURE 17 The long axial view. (Courtesy of Reilingh et al. [12]). (**a**) According to Lamm et al. [9], the patient is in the ski-jumping position (not pictured). The affected limb is in the centre of the film. The heel is closest to the edge of the film. The central ray is centred on the subtalar joint. The head of the tube is behind the affected limb and is inclined at a 45° angle to the vertical. (**b**) Radiograph showing the long axial view

jumping position: the affected ankle is in maximum dorsiflexion and the knee is extended. The affected limb is in the centre of the film and the unaffected limb is in front of the film. The heel is closest to the edge of the film. The central ray is centred on the subtalar joint. The head of the tube is behind the affected limb, 1.016 m from the heel, and is inclined at a 45° angle to the vertical [9].
- The angle between the mid-diaphyseal line of the tibia and the calcaneal bisection line is evaluated. The calcaneal bisection line (i.e. the frontal plane axis of the posterior heel) is obtained from the bisector of the radiographic silhouette of the calcaneus [9].
- Normal value: 2.1° of varus [9].
- It is not validated in children.

Bohler Angle

(Fig. 18, Table 7)
- Lines: from the posterior corner of the calcaneal apophysis to the proximal edge of the posterior facet/from the proximal edge of the posterior facet to the superior anterior aspect of the calcaneus at the calcaneocuboid joint [13].
- In the lateral view, with superimposition of both malleoli: 34° under the age of 5, 40° between 5 and 8 years of age and 33° between 13 and 16 years of age [14].
- It is used to assess the calcaneus deformity due to fracture; in particular, if the fracture involves the anterior process of the calcaneus, the angle decreases [2, 5].

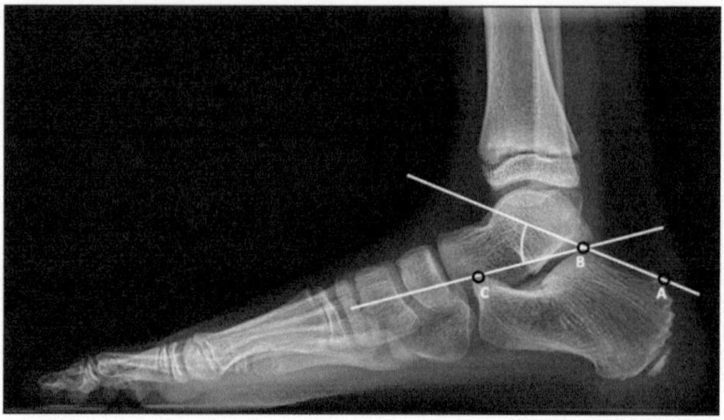

FIGURE 18 Bohler's angle. The angle between the lines drawn from the posterior corner of the calcaneal apophysis (*A*) to the proximal edge of the posterior facet (*B*) and from the proximal edge of the posterior facet (*B*) to the supero-anterior aspect of the calcaneus at the calcaneocuboid joint (*C*)

Gissane Angle

(Fig. 19, Table 7)

- Lines: posterior facet/middle facet.
- In the lateral view, with superimposition of both malleoli: 116° under the age of 5, 111° between 5 and 8 years of age and 110° between 13 and 16 years of age [14].
- It is used to assess the deformity of the calcaneus due to fracture [2, 5].

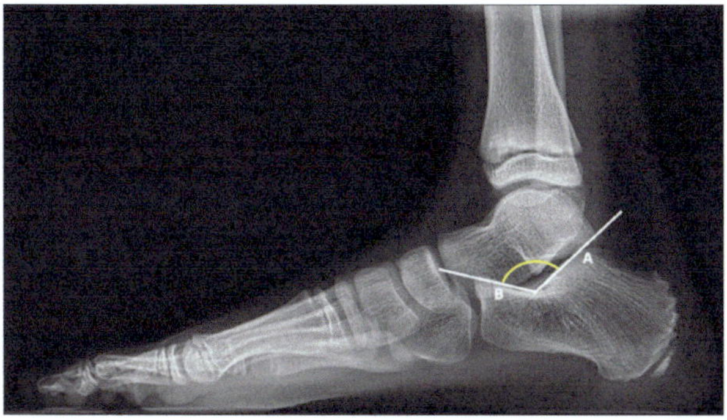

Figure 19 Gissane's angle. The angle between the posterior facet (*A*) and the middle facet (*B*) of the calcaneus

Table 7 Changes in Bohler and Gissane angles during growth (adapted from Pombo et al. [14])

Age (years)	Bohler angle (mean ± SD; °)	Gissane angle (mean ± SD; °)
0–4	33.6 ± 5.5	115.8 ± 7.3
5–8	39.7 ± 5.7	111.1 ± 7.5
9–12	35.1 ± 5.5	109.8 ± 7.2
13–16	33.0 ± 5.0	109.8 ± 7.1
0–16	35.4 ± 5.9	110.5 ± 7.4
≥18	31.7 ± 5.2	112.8 ± 7.4

SD standard deviation

Midfoot

Changes in hindfoot alignment are usually reflected in altered relationships between the hindfoot and midfoot. The navicular plays a pivotal role, yet it is the last bone to ossify. If it is not yet ossified, assessment of alignment depends on the metatarsal bases; the lateral cuneiform, which begins to ossify between the neonatal period and 19 months of age, may also help to indicate midfoot and hindfoot deformity.

In congenital clubfoot, ultrasonography is increasingly advocated for assessing deformity at birth and tracking treatment outcomes because it can visualise the cartilaginous attachments of the growing feet [15, 16].

To assess tarsal alignment, the tarsal joint surface angles can be measured on a lateral view; however, these measurements have not been validated in children.

The plantar arch is also best assessed in the lateral view by measuring the alignment of the hindfoot and metatarsals: the posterior portion of the arch is represented by the dorsally flexed calcaneus; the plantar angulation of the distal metatarsal bones forms the anterior portion of the arch. Several angles can be measured, including the Meary angle, the Djian-Annonier angle, the lateral calcaneus-fifth-metatarsal angle and the lateral calcaneus-first-metatarsal or Hibbs angle.

Ultrasound Measurements

(Fig. 20, Table 8)

- On medial view: in neutral position of the foot; by positioning the transducer at the medial border of the foot, in a slightly oblique position; a plane showing the medial malleolus, the lateral malleolus and the navicular is chosen.
  - The medial malleolus-navicular distance: the shortest distance between the medial malleolus and the medial part of the navicular:

    Normal value at birth: 8.5 ± 1.1 mm [17].

Decreased distance in congenital clubfoot (4.6 ± 1.7 mm) [15].

- The soft tissue thickness: the perpendicular distance from the skin surface to the medial border of the cartilaginous talus at the level of the midpoint of the ossification centre:

  Normal value at birth: 4.7 ± 0.7 mm [17].
  Increased thickness in congenital clubfoot (11.6 ± 2.0 mm) [15].

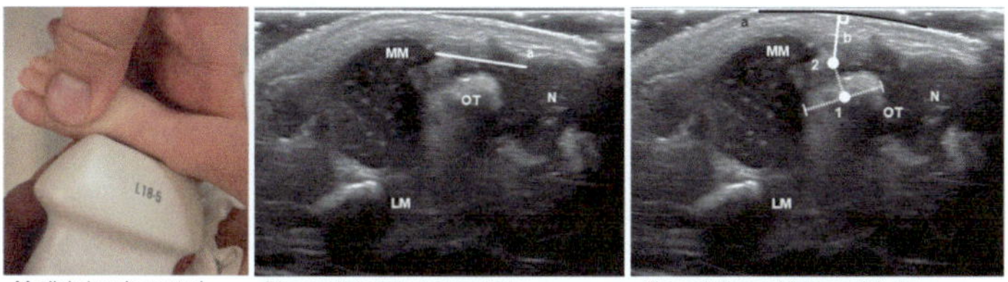

Medial view: in neutral position of the foot; by positioning the transducer at the medial border of the foot, in a slightly oblique position; a plane showing the medial malleolus, the lateral malleolus and the navicular is chosen.

The medial malleolus-navicular distance (*a*): the shortest distance between the medial malleolus (*MM*) and the medial part of the navicular (*N*).

OT: ossification centre of the talus
LM: lateral malleolus

The soft tissue thickness (*b*): the perpendicular distance from the skin surface (black line, *a*) to the medial border of the cartilaginous talus (dot *2*) at the level of the mid-point (dot *1*) of the ossification centre (*OT*).

N: navicular
LM: lateral malleolus
MM: medial malleolus

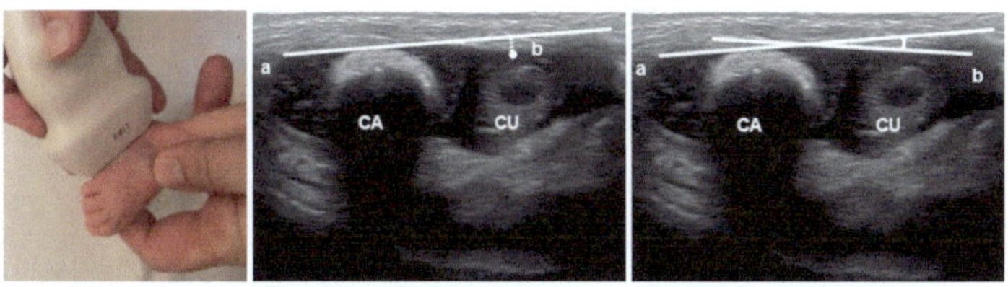

Lateral view: in neutral position of the foot; by positioning the transducer at the lateral border of the foot, parallel to the plantar aspect of the foot.

The calcaneocuboid distance: the perpendicular distance (dotted line, *b*) between the tangent along the lateral border of the calcaneus (*a*) and the mid-point (white dot) of the lateral cartilage border of the cuboid.

CA: calcaneus
CU: cuboid

The calcaneal-cuboid angle: formed by the lines tangential to the calcaneal body (*a*) and the cuboid (*b*).

CA: calcaneus
CU: cuboid

FIGURE 20 Ultrasound measurements

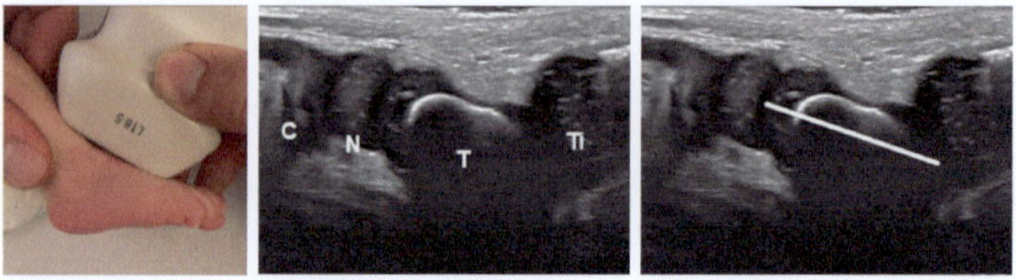

Dorsal view: in maximal plantar flexion; by positioning the transducer at the dorsal aspect of the foot.

In normal feet, the distal tibia (*Ti*), talus (*T*), navicular (*N*), first cuneiform (*C*) and first metatarsal bone are aligned.

The talus length.

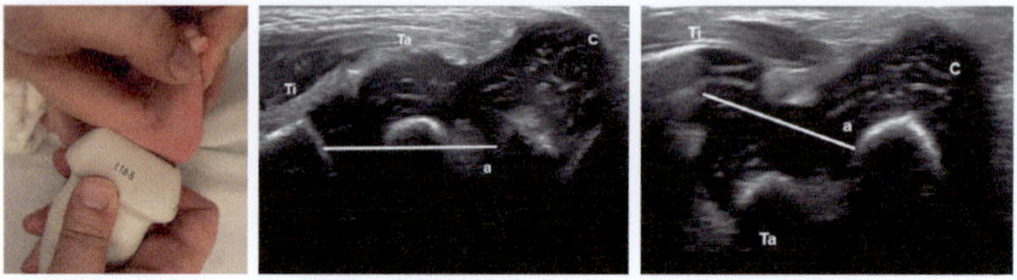

Sagittal posterior view: in plantar flexion and maximal dorsiflexion (as in the picture); by positioning the transducer vertically on the posterior border of the Achilles tendon.

Position of maximal dorsiflexion.

The tibiocalcaneal distance: the distance (*a*) between the distal tibial (*Ti*) metaphysis and the ossification centre of the calcaneus (*C*).

NB. The talus (*Ta*) is visualised into the ankle mortise.

Position of plantar flexion.

The tibiocalcaneal distance: the distance (*a*) between the distal tibial (*Ti*) metaphysis and the ossification centre of the calcaneus (*C*).

NB. The talus (*Ta*) is visualised anterior to the ankle mortise.

FIGURE 20 (continued)

- On lateral view: in neutral position of the foot; by positioning the transducer at the lateral border of the foot, parallel to the plantar aspect of the foot:
  - The calcaneocuboid distance: the perpendicular distance between the tangent along the lateral border of the calcaneus and the midpoint of the lateral cartilage border of the cuboid:

    Normal value at birth: 1.16 ± 1.1 mm [17].
    Increased distance in congenital clubfoot (2.5 ± 1.3 mm) [15].
  - The calcaneal-cuboid angle: formed by the lines tangential to the calcaneal body and the cuboid:

    Normal value: <12° [16]. (Newborn: <45 days).
    Increased angle in congenital clubfoot: mean 20° (range 16–32°) [16]. (Newborn: <45 days).

Table 8 Changes in ultrasound measurements of the infant's foot during growth (adapted from Aurell et al. [15])

Age (months)	Medial malleolus-navicular distance (mean ± SD; mm)	Calcaneocuboid distance (mean ± SD; mm)	Soft tissue thickness (mean ± SD; mm)	Length of talus (mean ± SD; mm)
0	8.5 ± 1.1	1.16 ± 1.1	4.7 ± 0.7	17.7 ± 1.1
4	9.7 ± 1.3	2.1 ± 1.2	5.5 ± 1.0	21.0 ± 1.3
7	10.8 ± 1.3	3.0 ± 1.1	6.2 ± 1.3	23.1 ± 1.6
12	12.3 ± 1.3	2.8 ± 1.3	7.6 ± 1.0	–

SD standard deviation

On dorsal view: in maximal plantar flexion; by positioning the transducer at the dorsal aspect of the foot. In normal feet, the talus, navicular, first cuneiform and first metatarsal bone are aligned. In clubfoot, the navicular is medially displaced [16].

- The talus length:

  Normal value at birth: 17.7 ± 1.1 mm [17].
  Decreased length in congenital clubfoot (14.5 ± 1.2 mm) [15].

- On sagittal posterior projection: in plantar flexion and maximal dorsiflexion; by positioning the transducer vertically on the posterior border of the Achilles tendon:
  - The tibiocalcaneal distance: the distance between the distal tibial metaphysis and the calcaneal apophysis:

    Normal values: mean 10 mm (range 8.5–12.5 mm) in plantar flexion; mean 20 mm (range 15–23 mm) in maximal dorsiflexion [16]. (Newborn: <45 days old).
    Decreased distance in maximal dorsiflexion in congenital clubfoot: mean 10.5 mm (range 9.5–11.5 mm) [16] (Newborn: <45 days old).

Lateral Tarsal Joint Surface Angles

(Fig. 21)

- Lines: parallel to the floor/lines drawn through the tarsal articular surfaces.
- In the lateral view, the articular surfaces of the talonavicular, the navicular-cuneiform and the first tarsometatarsal joints should show an approximately parallel alignment.
- The following normal ranges have been reported:
  - Talonavicular joint: 54–74°.
  - Navicular-cuneiform joint: 51–68°.
  - First tarsometatarsal joint: 55–72°.
- It is not validated in children.

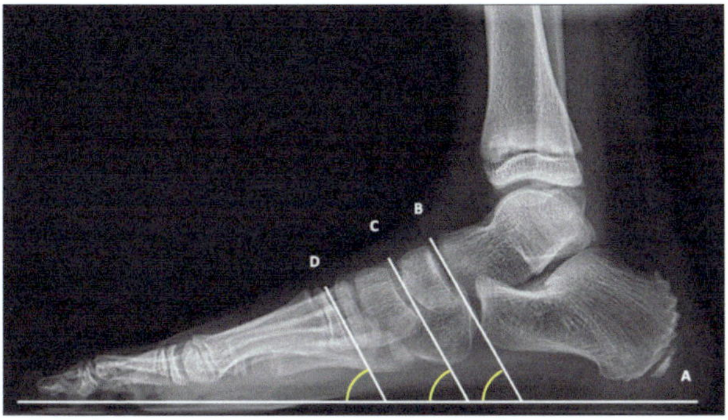

FIGURE 21 Lateral Tarsal joint surface angles. The angles between the parallel to the ground floor (*A*) and the lines drawn through the tarsal articular surfaces: (*B*) line through talonavicular joint, (*C*) line through naviculocuneiform joint, (*D*) line through first tarsometatarsal joint

Lateral Talar-First Metatarsal or Meary Angle

(Fig. 22, Table 9)

- Lines: midtalar line/first metatarsal shaft (the first metatarsal is easily distinguished as the shortest widest metatarsal).
- In the lateral view: near 0°; 19° (−2°; 40°) in the newborn and 8° (−5°; 21°) by age 4 years.
- Positive angles (usually >4° [2]) denote pes planus.
- Negative angles (usually < −4° [2]) denote pes cavus.

Djian-Annonier Angle

(Fig. 23)

- The angle between the most inferior point of the calcaneus, the most inferior point of the talonavicular joint and the most inferior point of the medial sesamoid (not visible in young children).

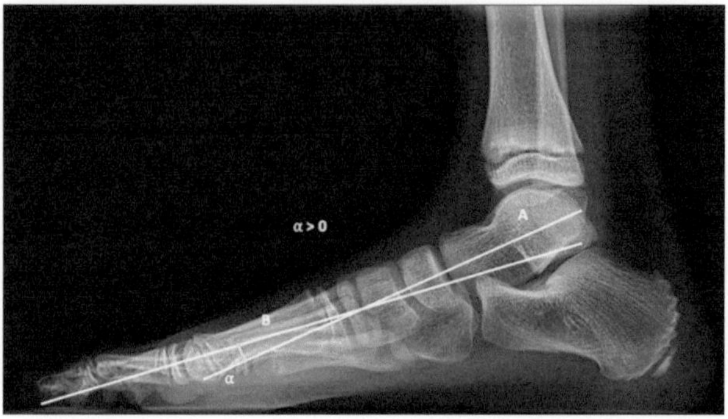

FIGURE 22 Talar-first metatarsal or Meary angle. The angle between the midtalar line (*A*) and the first metatarsal shaft (*B*). Positive angles denote a pes planus. Negative angles denote a pes cavus

TABLE 9 Changes in lateral weight-bearing talar / first metatarsal angle during growth (adapted from Vanderwilde et al. [10])

Age (years)	Mean (°)	−2SD (°)	+2SD (°)
0	18.5	−2.4	40.2
1	15.7	−3.6	34.2
2	12.4	−3.7	29.0
3	10.1	−4.9	24.3
4	8.3	−5.4	21.1
5	6.9	−5.7	19.8
6	5.6	−6.3	17.6
7	5.6	−6.6	17.2
8	5.6	−6.4	17.4
9	5.2	−6.9	18.9

Positive angles denote a planovalgus posture
SD standard deviation

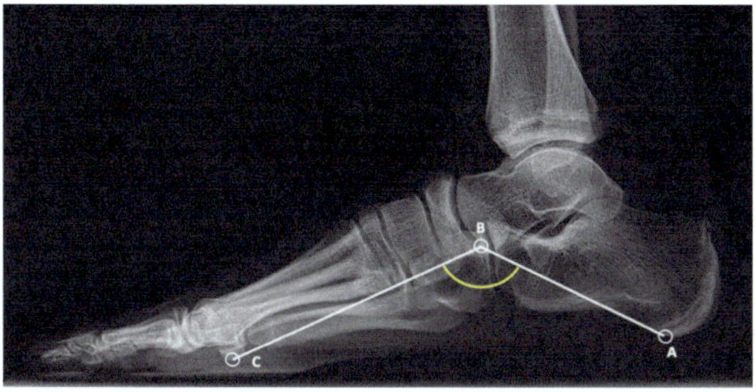

FIGURE 23 Djian-Annonier angle. The angle between the most inferior point of the calcaneus (*A*), the most inferior point of the talonavicular joint (*B*) and the most inferior point of the medial sesamoid (*C*)

- In the lateral view, normal values: 120°–130° [7, 18].
- Angles >130° denote a pes planus [7, 18].
- Angles <120° denote a pes cavus [7, 18].
- It's not validated in children.

Lateral Calcaneus-Fifth Metatarsal Angle

(Fig. 24)

- Lines: tangent to the inferior border of the calcaneus/fifth metatarsal shaft.
- In the lateral view: between 150° and 175° (apex upward) [2].
- A reduced angle with apex upward is observed in pes cavus [2].
- An excessive angle with apex upward is observed in pes planus [2].
- An excessive angle with apex downward is observed in congenital equinovarus and rocker bottom deformity [2].

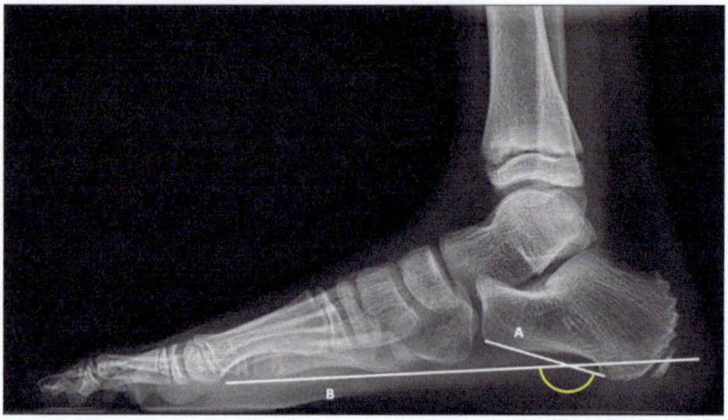

FIGURE 24 Lateral Calcaneus-fifth metatarsal angle. The angle between the tangents to the inferior border of the calcaneus (*A*) and the fifth metatarsal shaft (*B*)

Lateral Calcaneus-First Metatarsal or Hibbs Angle

(Fig. 25)

- Lines: midcalcaneal/first metatarsal shaft.
- In the lateral view: 150° [1].
- A reduced angle (usually <140° [1]) is observed in pes cavus.

Forefoot

Relative metatarsal lengths can be assessed using various methods such as the metatarsal index, Morton's method, Hardy and Clapham's method and metatarsal depth angle; however, these methods have not been validated in children.

Forefoot adduction and abduction describe the metatarsal position solely in the plane of the foot, without inversion or eversion of the plantar surface. In an AP projection, the metatarsals essentially move as a unit toward (adduction) or away from (abduction) the midline, pivoting at their bases; in a

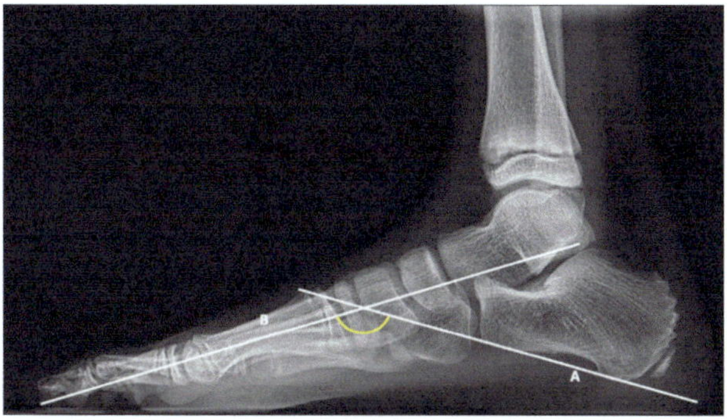

Figure 25 Lateral Calcaneus-first metatarsal or Hibbs angle. The angle between the midcalcaneal line (*A*) and the first metatarsal shaft (*B*)

lateral projection, the normal superimposition of the central metatarsals is maintained (unless there is an associated inversion or eversion).

Inversion and eversion are complex deformities of the entire foot.

Inversion combines supination, adduction and plantar flexion: in the AP view, metatarsal bases are superimposed and distal metatarsals swing toward the midline; in the lateral view, a ladder-like array may be seen, with the fifth metatarsal more plantar than the first one.

Eversion combines pronation, abduction and dorsiflexion: in the AP view, there is increased separation of the metatarsal bases and the metatarsal shafts are more parallel and less divergent; in the lateral view, a ladder-like array may be seen, with the first metatarsal more plantar than the fifth.

The relationship between metatarsals can be evaluated through the metatarsus adductus angle, the modified metatarsus adductus angle, the angle between the long axes of the calcaneus and the second metatarsal, the AP talar-first metatarsal angle and the AP calcaneal-fifth metatarsal angle.

Also, the presence of hallux valgus has to be evaluated.

Metatarsal Index

(Fig. 26)

- Line: uniform arc across the distal ends of the second through the fifth metatarsal.

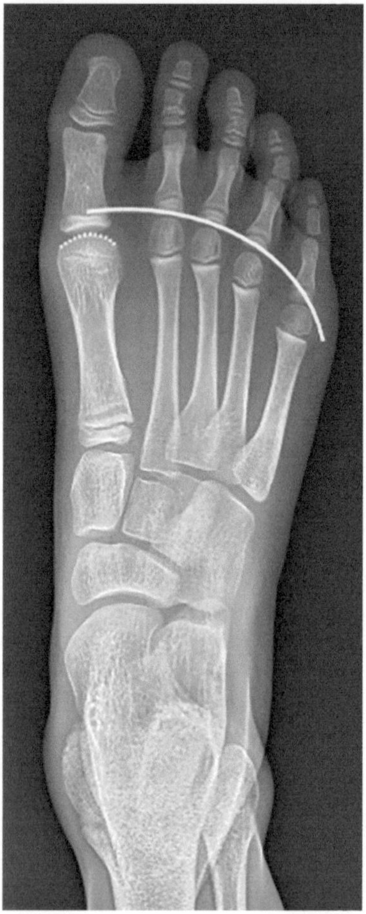

FIGURE 26 Metatarsal index. The relationship between the head of the first metatarsal (dotted line) and a uniform arc across the distal ends of the second through the fifth metatarsal (continuous line). In this picture, we observe a minus index: the first metatarsal head is proximal to the arc

- In the AP view, observing the relationship between the head of the first metatarsal and the line, we can distinguish:
  - Plus index: the first metatarsal head is distal to the arc.
  - Plus-minus index: the distal end of the first metatarsal head touches the arc.
  - Minus index: the first metatarsal head is proximal to the arc.
- A minus index indicates a predisposition to hallux valgus and metatarsalgia [2].
- It is not validated in children.

Morton's Method

(Fig. 27)

- Line: perpendicular to the longitudinal axis of the second metatarsal, through the head of the second metatarsal.
- On AP view, observing the relationship between the head of the first metatarsal and the line, we can distinguish:
  - Plus rating: horizontal line extends proximal (> 2 mm) to first metatarsal head (long first metatarsal).
  - Minus rating: horizontal line extends distal (>2 mm) to first metatarsal head (short first metatarsal) [19].
- A valgus or varus deformity of the first ray can distort the measurements.
- It is not validated in children.

Hardy and Clapham's Method

(Fig. 28)

- Lines: the axes of the first and second metatarsals are drawn; a transverse tarsal line is drawn to touch the posterior articular surface of the cuboid and the posterior aspect of the tuberosity of the navicular. At the point of intersection of this line with the axis of the second meta-

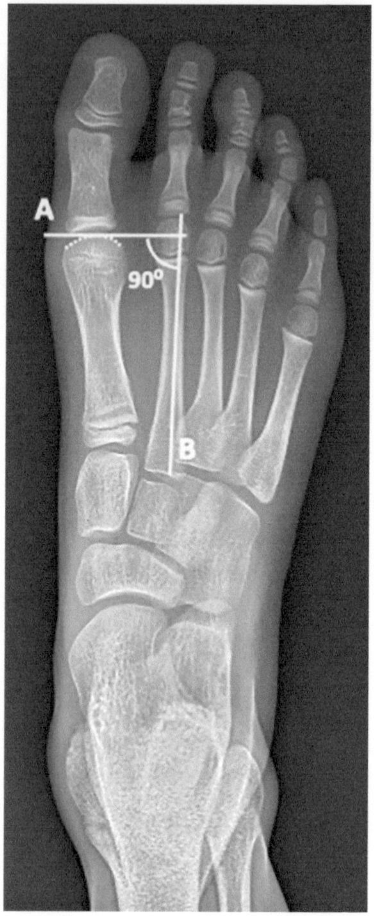

FIGURE 27 Morton's method. Based on the relationship between the head of the first metatarsal (dotted line) and a reference line (*A*), perpendicular to the longitudinal axis of the second metatarsal (*B*), through the head of the second metatarsal. We can distinguish: Plus rating: horizontal line extends proximal to first metatarsal head (long first metatarsal); Minus rating: horizontal line extends distal to first metatarsal head (short first metatarsal)

tarsal (point Z), the point of a pair of dividers is placed; arcs are then drawn to touch the articular surfaces of the heads of the first and second metatarsals.

- In the AP view, the radial distance (in mm) between the arcs is taken as the measure of relative metatarsal protrusion: a positive sign indicates that the first is greater than

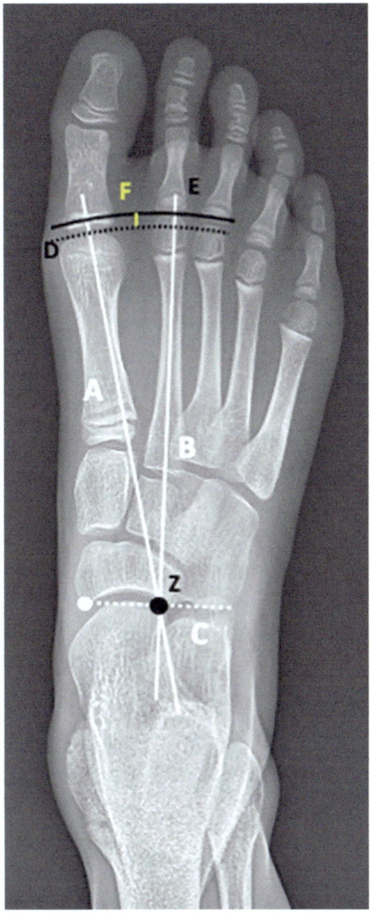

FIGURE 28 Hardy and Clapham's method. The axes of the first (*A*) and second (*B*) metatarsals are drawn; a transverse tarsal line (*C*) is drawn to touch the posterior articular surface of the cuboid and the posterior aspect of the tuberosity of the navicular (white dot). At the point of intersection of this line with the axis of the second metatarsal (black dot, *z*), the center of rotation is placed; arcs are then drawn to touch the articular surfaces of the heads of the first (*D*, dotted black curved line) and second (*E*, bold black curved line) metatarsals. The radial distance (*F*) between the arcs is taken as the measure of relative metatarsal protrusion. In this picture, a negative sign indicates that the second metatarsal is greater than the first

the second; a negative sign that the second is greater than the first.

- In the cases of hallux valgus, the first metatarsal is longer (>2 mm) than in the controls [20].
- It is not validated in children.

Metatarsal Depth Angle

(Fig. 29)

- Lines: tangent to the first and the second metatarsal heads/ tangent to the second and the fifth metatarsal heads.
- In the AP view: 142.5°.

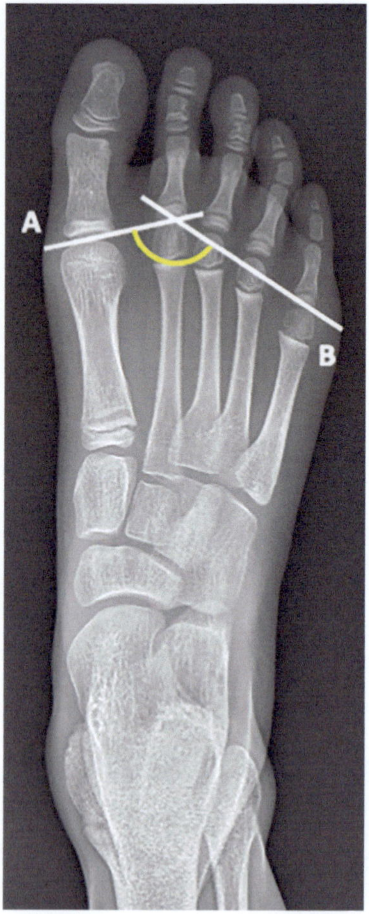

FIGURE 29 Metatarsal depth angle. The angle between the tangent to the first and the second metatarsal heads (*A*) and the tangent to the second and the fifth metatarsal heads (*B*)

- If the angle is <135°, a relative shortening of the first metatarsal can be denoted [2, 21].
- It is not validated in children.

Metatarsus Adductus Angle

(Fig. 30)

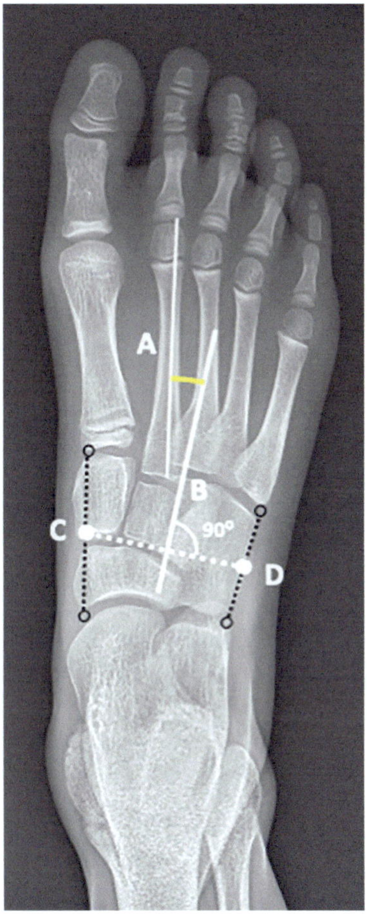

FIGURE 30 Metatarsus adductus angle. The angle between the axis of the second metatarsal (*A*) and the perpendicular (*B*) to a line drawn between the midpoint (*C*) between the medial aspect of the first metatarsal-cuneiform joint and the medial aspect of the talonavicular joint; and the midpoint (*D*) between the lateral aspect of the fifth metatarsal-cuboid joint and the lateral aspect of the calcaneocuboid joint

- Lines: axis of the second metatarsal/perpendicular to a line AB, where:
  - A is the midpoint between the medial aspect of the first metatarsal-cuneiform joint and the medial aspect of the talonavicular joint.
  - B is the midpoint between the lateral aspect of the fifth metatarsal-cuboid joint and the lateral aspect of the calcaneocuboid joint.
- Useful only in children whose tarsal bones are mostly ossified.
- In the AP view: between 10° and 20° [2, 5].
- An excessive angle is observed in forefoot adduction [5].

Modified Metatarsus Adductus Angle or Engel's Method

(Fig. 31)
- Lines: axis of the second metatarsal/axis of the medial cuneiform.
- Useful only in children whose tarsal bones are mostly ossified.
- In the AP view: between 13° and 23° [22].
- An excessive angle is observed in forefoot adduction [5].

Angle Between Calcaneus and Second Metatarsal

(Fig. 32)
- Lines: midcalcaneal/second metatarsal axis.
- In the AP view: ≤ 22° (mean value 10°) [2].
- It is usually used in newborns and small children when the tarsal bones are not yet fully ossified and the metatarsus adducts angle evaluation can be challenging.
- An excessive angle is observed in forefoot adduction.

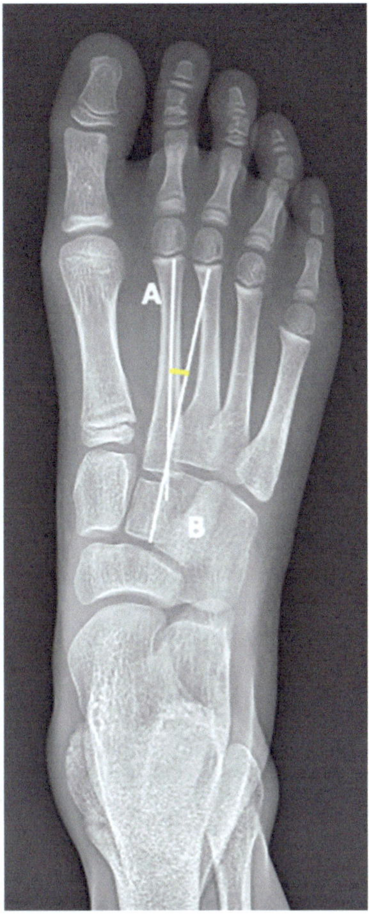

FIGURE 31 Modified metatarsus adductus angle or Engel's method. The angle between the axis of the second metatarsal (*A*) and the axis of the medial cuneiform (*B*)

AP Talar-First Metatarsal Angle

(Fig. 33, Table 10)

- Lines: midtalar/first metatarsal axis.
- In the AP view: 21° (9°; 31°) in the newborn and 10° (−4°; 24°) by age 4 years [10].

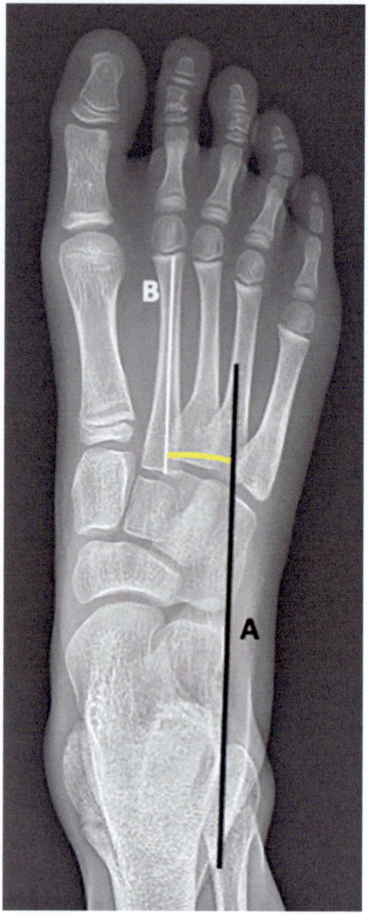

FIGURE 32 Angle between calcaneus and second metatarsal. The angle between the midcalcaneal line (*A*) and the second metatarsal axis (*B*)

- The angle usually is between 0° and 20°. A negative angle, with lateral positioning of the midtalar line, can be observed in forefoot adduction and clubfoot [11].
- NB: Simons et al. [11] consider positive angle as pathological and negative as physiological. We used a different definition to be consistent with measurements given by Vanderwilde et al. [10].

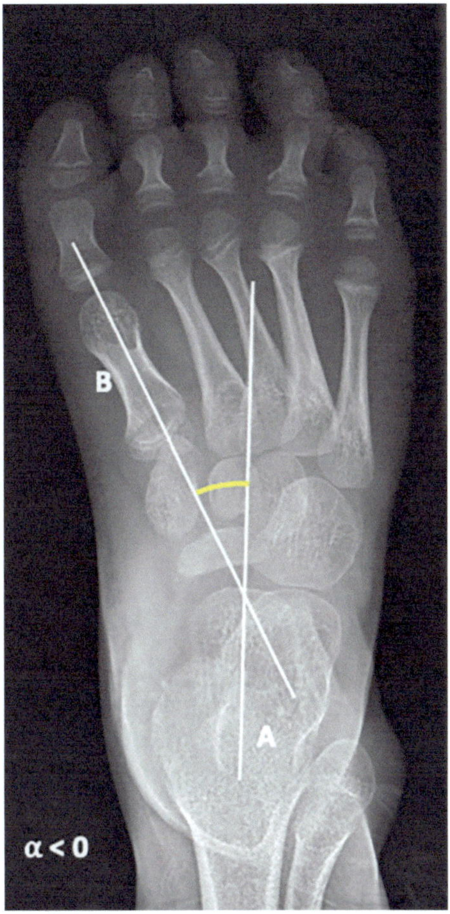

FIGURE 33 AP Talar-first metatarsal angle. The angle between the midtalar line (*A*) and the first metatarsal axis (*B*). In the picture a negative angle, with lateral positioning of the midtalar line, can be observed

TABLE 10 Changes in AP weight-bearing talar-first metatarsal angle during growth (adapted from Vanderwilde et al. [10])

Age (years)	Mean (°)	−2SD (°)	+2SD (°)
0	20.5	9.1	31.4
1	16.8	5.2	29.5
2	14.6	1.6	27.0
3	12.2	−0.9	25.2
4	10.4	−3.6	23.8
5	8.4	−5.7	22.2
6	6.6	−7.2	20.7
7	5.5	−8.1	19.3
8	3.9	−9.0	18.3
9	3.2	−9.7	17.3

SD standard deviation

AP Calcaneal-Fifth Metatarsal Angle

(Fig. 34, Table 11)

- Lines: midcalcaneal/fifth metatarsal axis.
- In the AP view: 2 (−9°; 15°) in the newborn, −1 (−10°; −9°) by age 4 years and then increasing [10].
- Positive angles indicate that the distal projection of the fifth metatarsal is directed more laterally than the axis of the calcaneus.
- Angles can be disturbed in metatarsus adductus [5].

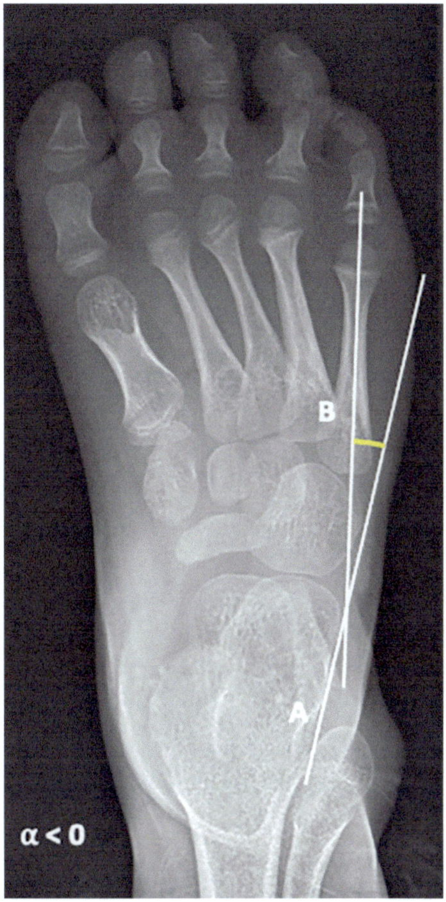

FIGURE 34 AP Calcaneal-fifth metatarsal angle. The angle between the midcalcaneal line (*A*) and the fifth metatarsal axis (*B*). Positive angles indicate that the distal projection of the fifth metatarsal is directed more laterally than the axis of the calcaneus. In the picture, a negative angle indicates that the distal projection of the fifth metatarsal is directed more medially than the axis of the calcaneus

TABLE 11 Changes in AP weight-bearing calcaneal-fifth metatarsal angle during growth (adapted from Vanderwilde et al. [10])

Age (years)	Mean (°)	–2SD (°)	+2SD (°)
0	2.4	–9.1	14.6
1	0.9	–9.9	11.9
2	–0.4	–10.0	9.9
3	–0.8	–10.2	8.9
4	–1.3	–10.2	8.3
5	–1.2	–10.1	8.5
6	–0.5	–9.9	9.0
7	0.3	–9.1	10.5
8	2.0	–8.8	13.0
9	3.8	–7.4	15.1

SD standard deviation

Hallux Valgus Angle

(Fig. 35)

- Lines: proximal phalanx axis of the first ray/first metatarsal axis.
- In the AP view: 8° ± 3°.
- A hallux valgus angle greater than 15° is considered pathological [23].

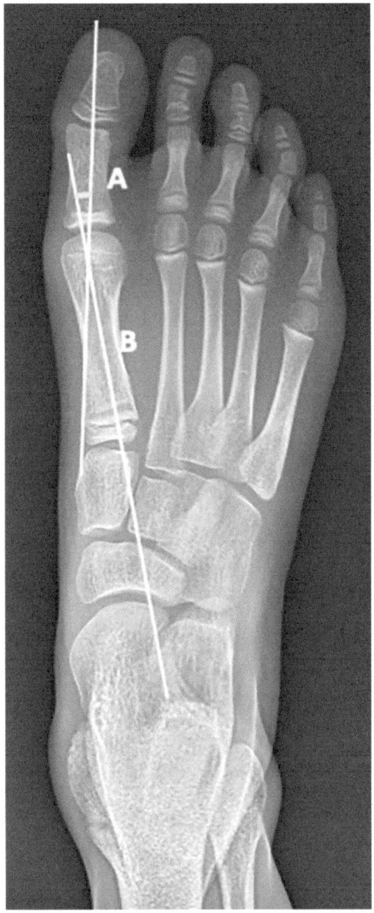

Figure 35 Hallux valgus angle. The angle between the proximal phalanx axis of the first ray (*A*) and the first metatarsal axis (*B*)

References

1. Stein-Wexler R, Wootton-Gorges SL, Ozonoff MB. Pediatric orthopedic imaging. Berlin, Heidelberg: Springer-Verlag; 2015. https://www.springer.com/gp/book/9783642453809.
2. Waldt S, Woertler K. Measurements and classifications in musculoskeletal radiology. New York: Thieme Verlag; 2014. https://www.thieme-connect.de/products/ebooks/book/10.1055/b-002-91661. Accessed 31 Aug 2021.
3. Paley D. Principles of deformity correction. Berlin: Springer Science & Business Media; 2002. p. 860.
4. Paley D, Herzenberg JE, Tetsworth K, McKie J, Bhave A. Deformity planning for frontal and sagittal plane corrective osteotomies. Orthop Clin North Am. 1994;25(3):425–65.
5. Cassar-Pullicino VN, Davies AM, editors. Measurements in musculoskeletal radiology. Berlin, Heidelberg: Springer-Verlag; 2020. (Diagnostic Imaging). https://www.springer.com/gp/book/9783540438533. Accessed 31 Aug 2021.
6. Neri T, Barthelemy R, Tourné Y. Analyse radiologique de l'alignement de l'arrière-pied: comparaison entre les clichés de Meary, long axial view et hindfoot alignment view. Revue de Chirurgie Orthopédique et Traumatologique. 2017;103(8):882–7.
7. Serra-Tosio G. Repères et mesures utiles en imagerie ostéo-articulaire. Issy-les-Moulineaux: Elsevier-Masson; 2011. (Imagerie médicale, pratique).
8. Saltzman CL, El-Khoury GY. The hindfoot alignment view. Foot Ankle Int. 1995;16(9):572–6.
9. Lamm BM, Mendicino RW, Catanzariti AR, Hillstrom HJ. Static Rearfoot alignment: a comparison of clinical and radiographic measures. J Am Podiatr Med Assoc. 2005;95(1):26–33.
10. Vanderwilde R, Staheli LT, Chew DE, Malagon V. Measurements on radiographs of the foot in normal infants and children. J Bone Joint Surg Am. 1988;70(3):407–15.
11. Simons G. Analytical radiography of club feet. J Bone Joint Surg. 1977;59-B(4):485–9.
12. Reilingh ML, Beimers L, Tuijthof GJM, et al. Measuring hindfoot alignment radiographically: the long axial view is more reliable than the hindfoot alignment view. Skeletal Radiol. 2010;39:1103–8. https://doi.org/10.1007/s00256-009-0857-9.
13. Böhler L. Diagnosis, pathology, and treatment of fractures of the OS CALCIS. J Bone Jt Surg. 1931;13(1):75–89.

14. Pombo B, Ferreira AC, Costa L. Bohler angle and the crucial angle of Gissane in Paediatric population. Clin Med Insights Arthritis Musculoskelet Disord. 2019;12:1179544119835227.
15. Aurell Y, Johansson A, Hansson G, Jonsson K. Ultrasound anatomy in the neonatal clubfoot. Eur Radiol. 2002;12(10):2509–17.
16. Gigante C, Talenti E, Turra S. Sonographic assessment of clubfoot. J Clin Ultrasound. 2004;32(5):235–42.
17. Aurell Y, Johansson A, Hansson G, Wallander H, Jonsson K. Ultrasound anatomy in the normal neonatal and infant foot: an anatomic introduction to ultrasound assessment of foot deformities. Eur Radiol. 2002;12(9):2306–12.
18. Bouysset M. Pathologie ostéo-articulaire du pied et de la cheville: approche médico-chirurgicale. Berlin: Springer Science & Business Media; 2004. p. 602.
19. Karasick D, Wapner KL. Hallux valgus deformity: preoperative radiologic assessment. AJR Am J Roentgenol. 1990;155(1):119–23.
20. Hardy RH, Clapham JCR. Observations on hallux valgus; based on a controlled series. J Bone Joint Surg Br. 1951;33-B(3):376–91.
21. Gamble FO, Yale I. Clinical foot roentgenology. Malabar, FL: R. E. Krieger Publishing Company; 1975. p. 456.
22. Engel E, Erlick N, Krems I. A simplified metatarsus adductus angle. J Am Podiatry Assoc. 1983;73(12):620–8.
23. McCluney JG, Tinley P. Radiographic measurements of patients with juvenile hallux valgus compared with age-matched controls: a cohort investigation. J Foot Ankle Surg. 2006;45(3):161–7.

Body Composition

Paolo Simoni

Introduction

Body composition imaging (BCI) provides a quantitative assessment of body components such as fat, lean mass, and mineral bone [1]. Measurements can assess the whole body, but they can also be targeted to specific areas, such as the abdomen or lower limbs [2].

BCI is an important tool in clinical management of children and adolescents affected by overweight and obesity [3].

In addition, BCI can be used as a tool to evaluate the overall metabolic status of children and adolescents with eating disorders, endocrine pathologies, and other chronic diseases [4].

Abdominal fat content plays a key role in several metabolic pathways that can affect the long-term health of children and adolescents [5].

P. Simoni (✉)
Pediatric Imaging Department, Reine Fabiola Children's University Hospital, Université Libre de Bruxelles, Brussels, Belgium

P. Simoni, M. P. Aparisi Gómez (eds.), *Essential Measurements in Pediatric Musculoskeletal Imaging*,
https://doi.org/10.1007/978-3-031-17735-4_11

Abdominal fat (AF) can be broken down into subcutaneous fatty tissue (SAT) and visceral adipose fatty tissue (VAT), the latter having the greatest impact on metabolism [6].

Various imaging techniques have been used to assess body composition, including dual-energy X-ray absorptiometry (DXA), nuclear medicine, computed tomography (CT), magnetic resonance imaging (MRI), and ultrasound (US) [1]. Although most of the measurements discussed in this chapter are not yet performed in routine clinical practice, the rapid advances in the field of quantitative imaging and the steeply increasing rate of obese and overweight children and adolescents will require their use in routine clinical practice in the next future [2].

DXA and MRI have been better studied in the pediatric population and some normative values are presented in this chapter. The other imaging modalities need to be fully validated.

Given the variability of body composition estimates in children, including by age, gender, and ethnic group [7], quantification of any body composition parameter should also be related to individual patients by tracking changes during their treatment and follow-up.

Interestingly, CT can be used opportunistically in children when performed for other reasons, without supplementary irradiation, as body composition estimates on CT correlate well with those on MRI [8].

Advanced automated post-processing techniques are time-saving and promise to improve the reliability of BMI measurements [1].

DXA

DXA is a widely used technique to assess body composition in pediatric population [9].

In the past, DXA was only used to calculate the total and segmental bone mass density [10] (Fig. 1, left, in black and white).

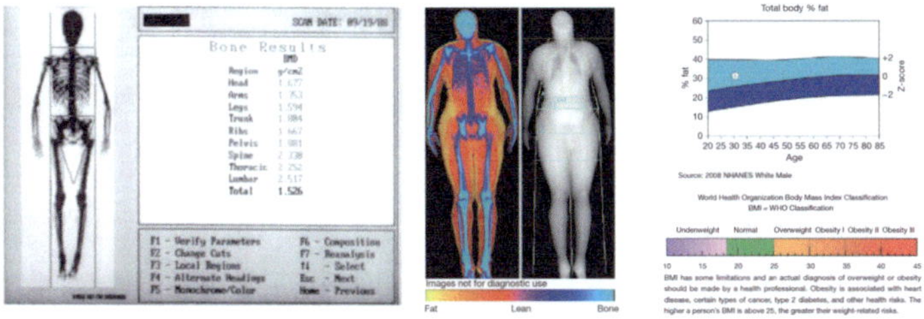

FIGURE 1 Example of body composition assessment in 1990 by DXA and a modern evaluation in 2016. (Reproduced with permission from Shepherd et al. [10])

Nowadays, DXA allows measuring the relative percentage of fat mass (FM), lean mass (LM), and mineral bone. It also offers the visual distribution of these compounds [10] (Fig. 1, right, in colors).

All components can be evaluated in a single individual and compared to those of the general population [2].

As a reminder, the *Z*-score represents the number of standard deviations away from the average value of the reference population, i.e.: *Z*-score = (patient's value − expected value)/standard of reference for the population.

The other measurements currently used in children and their acronyms along with the definition are the following [2]:

- Fat mass index (FMI) (kg/m^2): calculated as FM divided by $height^2$.
- Percentage of FM (% FM): calculated as FM (kg) divided by total body weight (kg).
- Trunk/limb fat ratio (FM trunk/limb): calculated as FM trunk divided by the sum of FM of arms and legs.
- Lean mass index (LMI) (kg/m^2): calculated as LM divided by $height^2$.
- Appendicular lean mass index (ALMI) (kg/m^2): the sum of LM of arms and of legs (appendicular lean mass - ALM) divided by $height^2$.
- Body mass index (BMI) (kg/m^2): calculated as body weight divided by $height^2$.
- Fitted FMI (kg/m): calculated as FM divided by height.

- Fitted LMI (kg/m): calculated as LM divided by height.
- Fitted ALMI (kg/m): calculated as ALM divided by height.
- Fitted BMI (kg/m): calculated as BM divided by height.

In children and adolescents, the values of SAT and VAT vary depending on the sex age and ethnic group [11] as shown in Fig. 2.

The general trends for the abdominal fat tissue distribution in adolescent after puberty are shown in Fig. 3.

Normative DXA values were recently provided studying a large population of European children and adolescents [11].

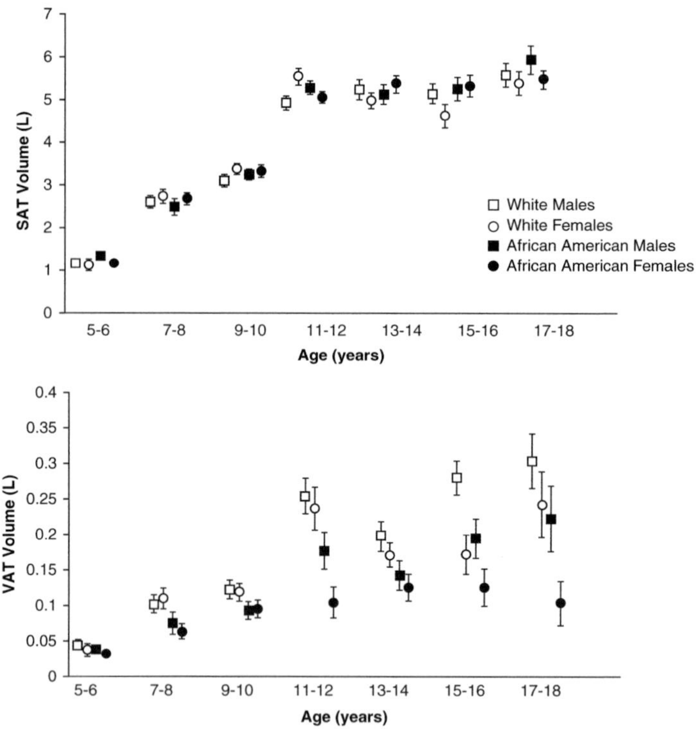

FIGURE 2 SAT and VAT plotted against age. (Reproduced with permission from Staiano et al. [11])

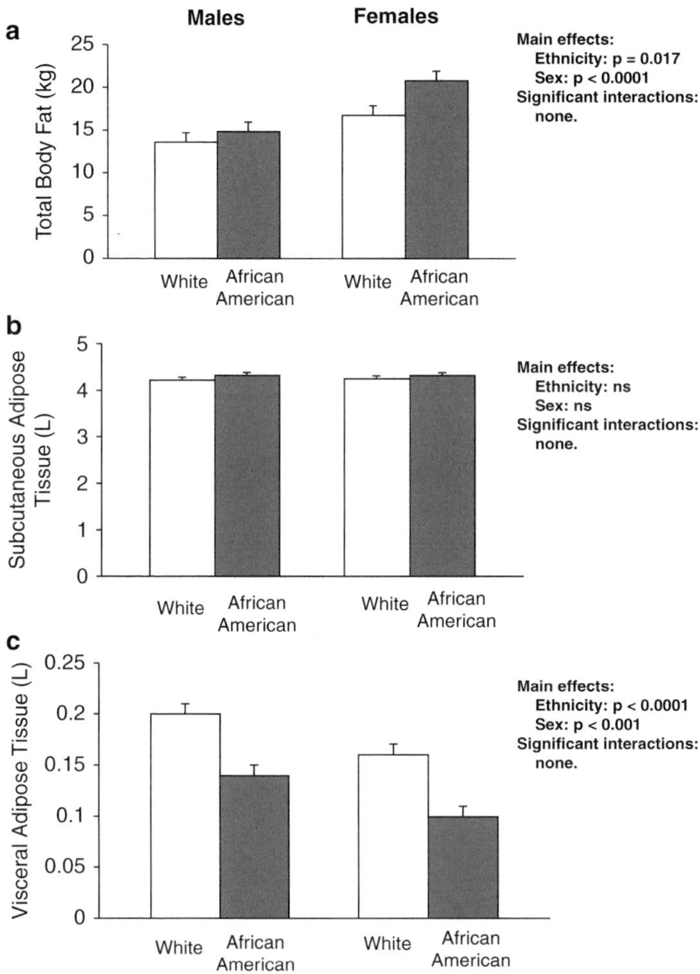

FIGURE 3 Abdominal fat tissue distribution in adolescents after puberty. (Reproduced with permission from Staiano et al. [11])

Hence, the reference values to calculate the *Z*-score for the whole body and for specific area are given in Table 1.

Graphics of BMI measurements plotted against the chronological age have also been provided. The curves allow calculating the percentile for a specific individual as shown in Fig. 4.

Table 1 Anthropometric and body composition normative value by class of age (Reproduced with permission from Ofenheimer et al. [2])

Age	6–18 years	6–8 years	8–10 years	10–12 years	12–14 years	14–16 years	16–18 years
Total							
Sample size (*n*)	1573	346	363	242	194	200	228
Height (cm)	147.3 ± 19.3	124.8 ± 6.4	135.3 ± 7.4	146.3 ± 7.8	160.2 ± 8.4	167.7 ± 8.4	172.5 ± 8.9
Weight (kg)	42.6 ± 17.7	25.3 ± 5.2	32.0 ± 7.7	39.7 ± 10.1	51.1 ± 11.6	60.6 ± 13.5	65.5 ± 11.1
BMI (kg/m^2)	18.7 ± 3.9	16.1 ± 2.3	17.3 ± 3.0	18.4 ± 3.6	19.8 ± 3.5	21.5 ± 4.3	22.0 ± 3.1
%FM	30.0 ± 7.9	29.8 ± 6.2	31.4 ± 7.8	31.6 ± 7.5	29.8 ± 8.2	30.1 ± 8.4	26.6 ± 8.5
FM (kg)	12.6 ± 7.1	7.5 ± 3.2	10.2 ± 4.9	12.7 ± 6.2	15.3 ± 7.2	18.1 ± 8.4	16.8 ± 6.7
LM (kg)	28.7 ± 12.0	17.1 ± 2.7	21.0 ± 3.6	25.9 ± 4.6	34.2 ± 6.4	40.5 ± 7.9	46.2 ± 8.9
ALM (kg)	12.9 ± 6.3	6.9 ± 1.5	8.9 ± 2.0	11.5 ± 2.4	15.8 ± 3.4	18.8 ± 4.4	21.9 ± 5.2
Males							
Sample size (*n*)	814	159	195	129	102	97	132
Height (cm)	149.6 ± 20.6	124.9 ± 6.5	135.9 ± 7.6	146.4 ± 7.5	161.0 ± 9.0	171.8 ± 8.7	177.5 ± 6.8
Weight (kg)	44.6 ± 19.1	25.6 ± 5.1	32.2 ± 8.1	40.3 ± 9.8	51.9 ± 12.0	64.4 ± 15.5	69.5 ± 10.4

BMI (kg/m²)	18.9 ± 4.0	16.3 ± 2.2	17.2 ± 3.0	18.7 ± 3.7	19.8 ± 3.4	21.8 ± 5.0	22.0 ± 2.9
%FM	27.2 ± 7.9	27.4 ± 5.7	28.9 ± 7.5	30.7 ± 7.8	27.8 ± 8.8	26.1 ± 8.9	21.3 ± 6.0
FM (kg)	11.8 ± 7.1	7.0 ± 2.8	9.5 ± 5.1	12.4 ± 6.4	14.5 ± 7.3	17.0 ± 9.8	14.5 ± 6.2
LM (kg)	31.2 ± 13.6	17.9 ± 2.7	21.8 ± 3.7	26.6 ± 4.2	35.7 ± 7.0	45.2 ± 8.3	52.1 ± 6.3
ALM (kg)	14.3 ± 7.2	7.2 ± 1.5	9.3 ± 2.1	11.9 ± 2.3	16.7 ± 3.8	21.5 ± 4.5	25.3 ± 3.8
Normal weight[a]	58%	61%	56%	51%	55%	56%	70%
Overweight[a]	18%	13%	20%	22%	24%	14%	15%
Obesity[a]	10%	12%	10%	13%	8%	13%	3%
Females							
Sample size (*n*)	759	187	168	113	92	103	96
Height (cm)	144.7 ± 17.4	124.7 ± 6.4	134.5 ± 7.0	146.1 ± 8.3	159.3 ± 7.6	163.8 ± 6.0	165.7 ± 6.7
Weight (kg)	40.4 ± 15.8	25.0 ± 5.4	31.8 ± 7.3	38.9 ± 10.4	50.2 ± 11.2	57.0 ± 10.2	60.1 ± 9.9
BMI (kg/m²)	18.5 ± 3.8	16.0 ± 2.3	17.4 ± 3.0	18.0 ± 3.6	19.7 ± 3.7	21.2 ± 3.6	21.9 ± 3.4
%FM	33.0 ± 6.5	31.8 ± 6.0	34.2 ± 7.2	32.7 ± 7.1	32.0 ± 7.0	33.8 ± 6.0	33.9 ± 5.7

(continued)

Table 1 (continued)

Age	6–18 years	6–8 years	8–10 years	10–12 years	12–14 years	14–16 years	16–18 years
FM (kg)	13.4 ± 7.0	8.0 ± 3.3	11.0 ± 4.6	12.9 ± 6.1	16.1 ± 7.0	19.2 ± 6.7	20.0 ± 6.2
LM (kg)	25.9 ± 9.2	16.5 ± 2.5	20.0 ± 3.4	25.0 ± 5.0	32.6 ± 5.3	36.1 ± 4.4	38.1 ± 4.9
ALM (kg)	11.4 ± 4.6	6.7 ± 1.4	8.5 ± 1.9	11.1 ± 2.6	14.8 ± 2.7	16.4 ± 2.5	17.2 ± 2.7
Normal weight[a]	60%	63%	52%	54%	61%	63%	71%
Overweight[a]	17%	16%	24%	14%	15%	19%	11%
Obesity[a]	7%	5%	11%	9%	4%	5%	5%

Note: Table shows mean ± SD or prevalence (%)
BMI body mass index, *%FM* percentage of fat mass, *FM* fat mass, *LM* lean mass, *ALM* appendicular lean mass
[a]Normal weight: *Z*-scores –1 to 1, overweight: *Z*-scores >1 to ≤2, obesity. *Z*-scores >2 (WHO 2007)

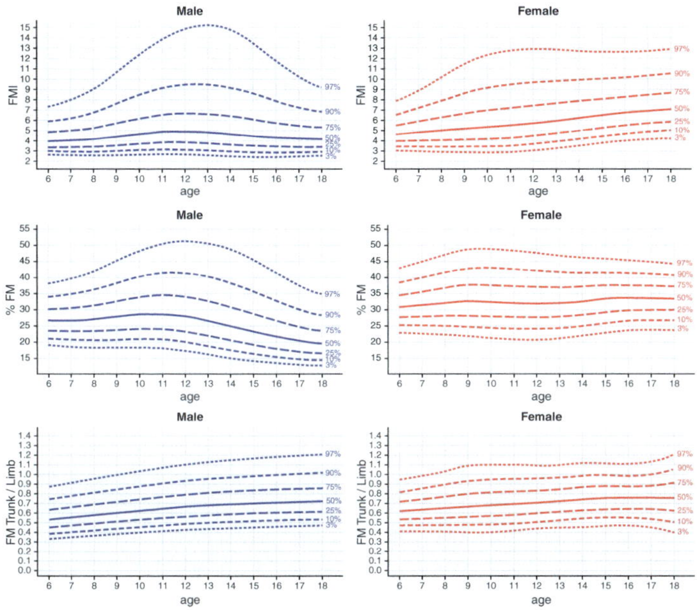

FIGURE 4 Fat mass index (FMI) percentage of fat mass (% FM) and trunk/limb fat ratio (FM trunk/limb) plotted against age. (Reproduced with permission from Ofenheimer et al. [2])

MRI

Magnetic resonance imaging allows to perform the same measurements described for DXA [12].

These measurements have not been not validated in a large population of children as those provided by DXA [13]. Normative values are limited to certain ages and ethnic groups.

However, in clinical practice, MRI allows to track the changes of the different body composition parameters over time in a patient without any radiation burden.

MRI enables to easily estimate VAT and SAT in terms of surface (cm^2) in both axial and coronal planes. Segmentation of contiguous planes can result in a more precise tridimensional evaluation.

The segmentation can be performed semiautomatically with free resource software, e.g., Horos (https://horosproject.org), using the "brushing tool" (Figs. 5 and 6).

Advanced software enables fast post-processing of the imaging [1].

Figures 7 and 8 show examples of fat and muscle automated quantitative segmentation: subcutaneous adipose tissue (light blue), visceral adipose tissue (red), right anterior thigh muscles (yellow), left anterior thigh muscles (pink), right posterior thigh-gluteal muscles (blue), and left posterior thigh-gluteal muscles (green).

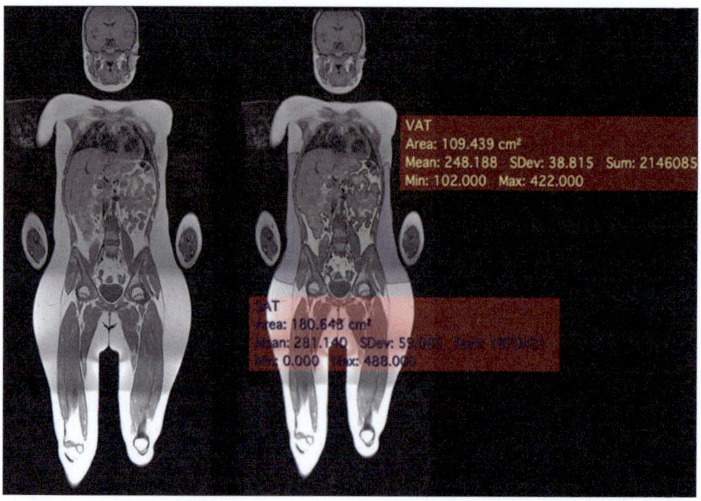

FIGURE 5 Segmentation performed semiautomatically with free resource software, e.g., Horos (https://horosproject.org) using the "brushing tool" on a whole-body MRI (assessment on a single coronal slice)

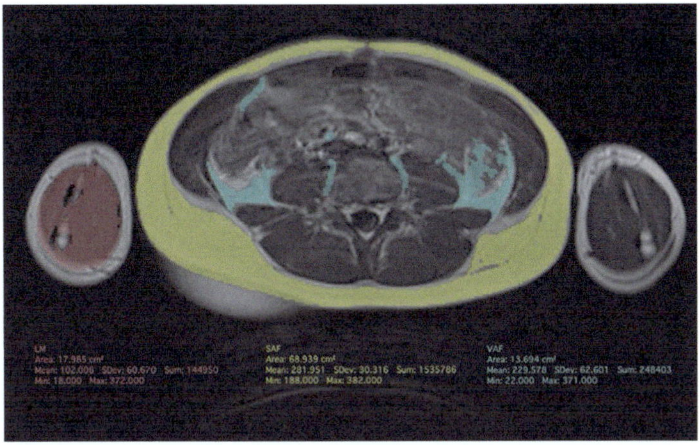

FIGURE 6 Segmentation performed semiautomatically with free resource software, e.g., Horos (https://horosproject.org) using the "brushing tool" on a single axial slice at the L3 level. The axial slice passing through the L3 vertebral body is considered to be a robust proxy to evaluate SAT and VAT of the whole abdomen

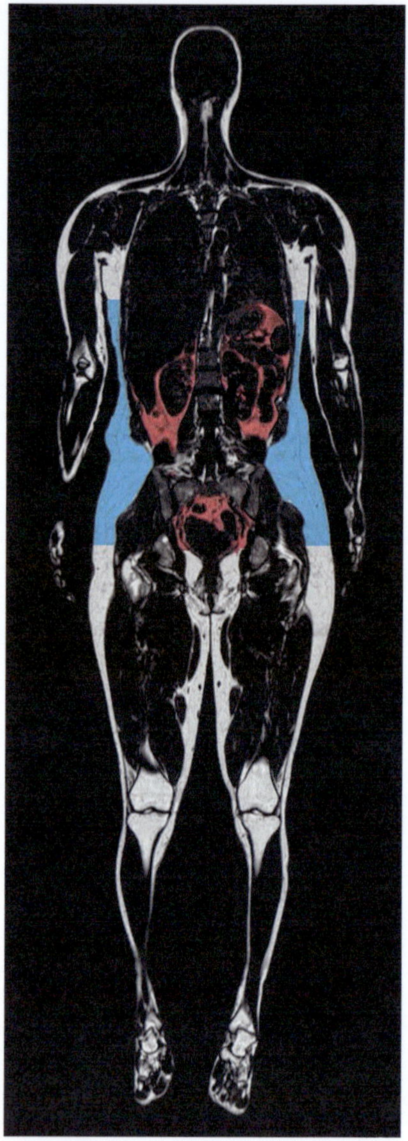

FIGURE 7 Example of an automatic segmentation of SAT and VAT on a whole-body MRI. (Courtesy of AMRA Medical—amramedical.com)

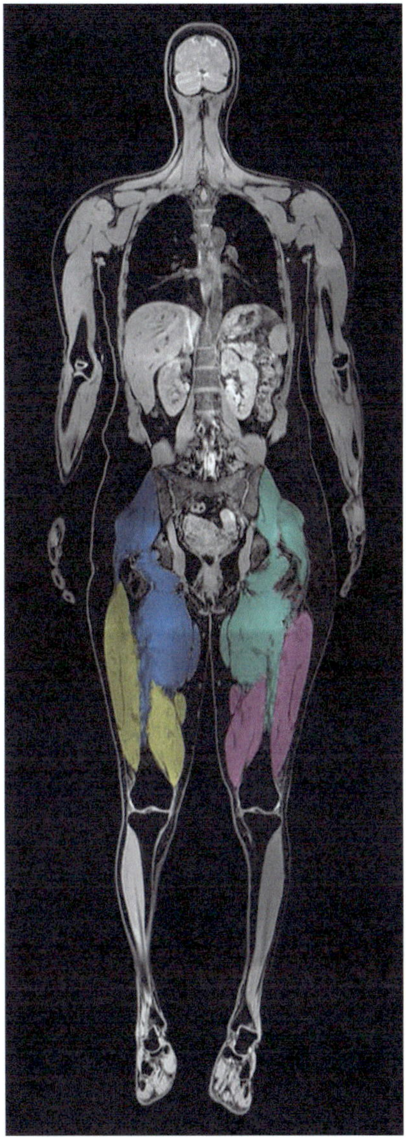

FIGURE 8 Example of an automatic segmentation of the muscles (lean mass) of the gluteal region and the thigh. A different color is used for each muscle group, with a side-to-side comparison, on a whole-body MRI. (Courtesy of AMRA Medical—amramedical.com)

References

1. Simoni P, Guglielmi R, Aparisi Gómez MP. Imaging of body composition in children. Quant Imaging Med Surg. 2020;10(8):1661–71.
2. Ofenheimer A, Breyer-Kohansal R, Hartl S, Burghuber OC, Krach F, Schrott A, et al. Reference charts for body composition parameters by dual-energy X-ray absorptiometry in European children and adolescents aged 6 to 18 years-results from the Austrian LEAD (lung, hEart, sociAl, boDy) cohort. Pediatr Obes. 2021;16(1):e12695.
3. Eloi JC, Epifanio M, de Goncalves MM, Pellicioli A, Vieira PF, Dias HB, et al. Quantification of abdominal fat in obese and healthy adolescents using 3 tesla magnetic resonance imaging and free software for image analysis. PLoS One. 2017;12(1):e0167625.
4. Haas VK, Kohn MR, Clarke SD, Allen JR, Madden S, Muller MJ, et al. Body composition changes in female adolescents with anorexia nervosa. Am J Clin Nutr. 2009;89(4):1005–10.
5. Llewellyn A, Simmonds M, Owen CG, Woolacott N. Childhood obesity as a predictor of morbidity in adulthood: a systematic review and meta-analysis. Obes Rev. 2016;17(1):56–67.
6. Kabir M, Catalano KJ, Ananthnarayan S, Kim SP, Van Citters GW, Dea MK, et al. Molecular evidence supporting the portal theory: a causative link between visceral adiposity and hepatic insulin resistance. Am J Physiol Endocrinol Metab. 2005;288(2):E454–61.
7. Satake E, Nakagawa Y, Kubota A, Saegusa H, Sano S, Ohzeki T. Age and sex differences in fat distribution in non-obese Japanese children. J Pediatr Endocrinol Metab. 2010;23(9):873–8.
8. Klopfenstein BJ, Kim MS, Krisky CM, Szumowski J, Rooney WD, Purnell JQ. Comparison of 3 T MRI and CT for the measurement of visceral and subcutaneous adipose tissue in humans. Br J Radiol. 2012;85(1018):e826–30.
9. Tagliabue L, Maioli C, Bonini M, Giacchero R. Measure of body composition by MOC DEXA, in children and teenagers with eating disorders. Prog Nutr. 2017;19(4):404–14.
10. Shepherd JA, Ng BK, Sommer MJ, Heymsfield SB. Body composition by DXA. Bone. 2017;104:101–5.

11. Staiano AE, Broyles ST, Gupta AK, Katzmarzyk PT. Ethnic and sex differences in visceral, subcutaneous, and total body fat in children and adolescents. Obesity (Silver Spring). 2013;21(6):1251–5.
12. Shearrer GE, House BT, Gallas MC, Luci JJ, Davis JN. Fat imaging via magnetic resonance imaging (MRI) in young children (ages 1-4 years) without sedation. PLoS One. 2016;11(2):e0149744.
13. Weber DR, Leonard MB, Zemel BS. Body composition analysis in the pediatric population. Pediatr Endocrinol Rev. 2012;10(1):130–9.

EOS Imaging

Alessandro De Leucio, Estelle Tenisch, Pierre Yves Zambelli, and Patrick Omoumi

Introduction

The EOS system is an X-ray system that allows to obtain high-quality whole-body radiograms with a much lower dose than conventional radiography in a standing or sitting position.

*A. De Leucio and E. Tenisch contributed equally.

A. De Leucio (✉)
Department of Radiology, Reine Fabiola University Children's Hospital, Brussels, Belgium
e-mail: alessandro.deleucio@huderf.be

E. Tenisch · P. Omoumi
Department of Diagnostic and Interventional Radiology, Lausanne University Hospital, Lausanne, Switzerland
e-mail: estelle.tenisch@chuv.ch

P. Y. Zambelli
Division of Pediatric Orthopedics, Department Women-mother-child, Lausanne University Hospital, Lausanne, Switzerland

P. Simoni, M. P. Aparisi Gómez (eds.), *Essential Measurements in Pediatric Musculoskeletal Imaging*,
https://doi.org/10.1007/978-3-031-17735-4_12

The technological key element of the EOS system is the multi-wire proportional chamber, for which Georges Charpak was awarded the Nobel Prize in 1992.

The high efficiency of the "Charpak chamber" to capture photons permits drastically lower milliampere (mA) values of the X-ray beam compared to traditional radiographic systems, resulting in high-quality diagnostic images obtained at very low doses [1–3].

Another significant technical element of EOS imaging is the very thinly collimated X-ray beam, which results almost parallel. Conventional radiographic systems use a conical X-ray beam that delivers a higher dose to the patient and induces the well-known magnification artifact for the structures far from the center of the image. The highly collimated parallel X-ray beam of the EOS system allows to reduce the dose and encounters only limited deformations of the images without magnification. Thus, EOS imaging is particularly suitable to obtain a 3D reconstruction of the spine and lower limb bony structures by stereoradiography [2, 4].

The EOS imaging system is composed of two X-ray tubes and two "Charpak's chambers," which move synchronously on the vertical axis, allowing the simultaneous acquisition of frontal and lateral images of the whole body. The possibility of obtaining images of the whole body and in a natural standing position makes the EOS system an excellent tool for studying pathologies of the spine, lower limbs, and pelvis in children and adults [3, 4].

The very low dose delivered to the patient is a highly valued element in pediatric radiology [1, 3].

After the acquisition, the EOS image undergoes advanced post-processing through the SterEOS® software [1, 2, 4].

SterEOS post-processing allows users to obtain a large number of measurements of medical interest automatically (whether scalar, vector, or angular) of the spine, pelvis, and lower limbs, in both a two-dimensional (2D) and three-dimensional (3D) way.

The EOS system is used for studying many pathologies of the lower limbs. EOS imaging allows an accurate assessment of lower limb length discrepancy, the deformation in varus or valgus, and many other pathologies, as well as being helpful for preoperative planning.

Usually, children can take the exam from the age when they can stand alone in the imaging system booth without moving for 40 s (generally from 7 years old in our experience).

Spine and Pelvis

Whenever available, low-dose radiography using EOS has replaced standard radiographs for the quantitative assessment of the spine and pelvis in children.

The following are a set of measurements routinely performed in clinical practice. The measurements may be performed using the SterEOS application or manually, using the software available on the PACS (Picture Archiving And Communication System).

Pelvic Measurements

Pelvic measurements are essential as the position of the pelvis determines the position of the lumbar spine and thereby of the entire spine. EOS imaging delivers a dose 2.4 inferior to conventional radiography when imaging the pelvis [5].

Pelvic Incidence (PI)

On the lateral view, the pelvic incidence (PI) is defined as the angle between two lines:

1. A line between the center of the femoral heads and the center of S1 endplate (if the femoral heads are not perfectly superposed on the lateral view, the reference point lies midway between the centers of the two femoral heads).
2. A line perpendicular to a line tangent to the endplate of S1.

The PI remains constant after skeletal maturity and does not change with the patient position. Pelvic incidence is the fundamental pelvic parameter in the three-dimensional development of the sagittal curves of the spine. Based on the PI value, the geometry of the physiological lumbar lordosis can be theoretically predicted [6].

The lower the PI, the narrower the pelvis (as measured in the anteroposterior axis). The greater the PI, the wider the pelvis. The PI increases slightly with age, following the onset of unassisted bipedal locomotion in children.

Normal values [7]:

- 44.0 ± 6.5 degrees in children between 2 and 9 years old.
- 48.1 ± 8.5 degrees in children between 10 and 15 years old.
- 46.6 ± 8.4 degrees in children between 15 and 20 years old (Fig. 1).

Sacral Slope (SS)

The sacral slope (SS) is defined as the angle between:

1. The horizontal plane.
2. The axis of S1 endplate.

The value of the SS may vary depending on the patient's position.

Hence, a horizontal pelvis has a greater SS and a vertically oriented pelvis has a lower SS value. The SS remains relatively unchanged during growth. Sagittal sacro-pelvic alignment is most commonly assessed in children from the pelvic tilt (PT) and the sacral slope (SS), i.e. PI=SS + PT.

Normal values [8]:

- Between 3 and 8 years old: 38.2 ± 7.7 °.
- Between 8 and 18 years old: 39.1 ± 7.6 ° (Fig. 2).

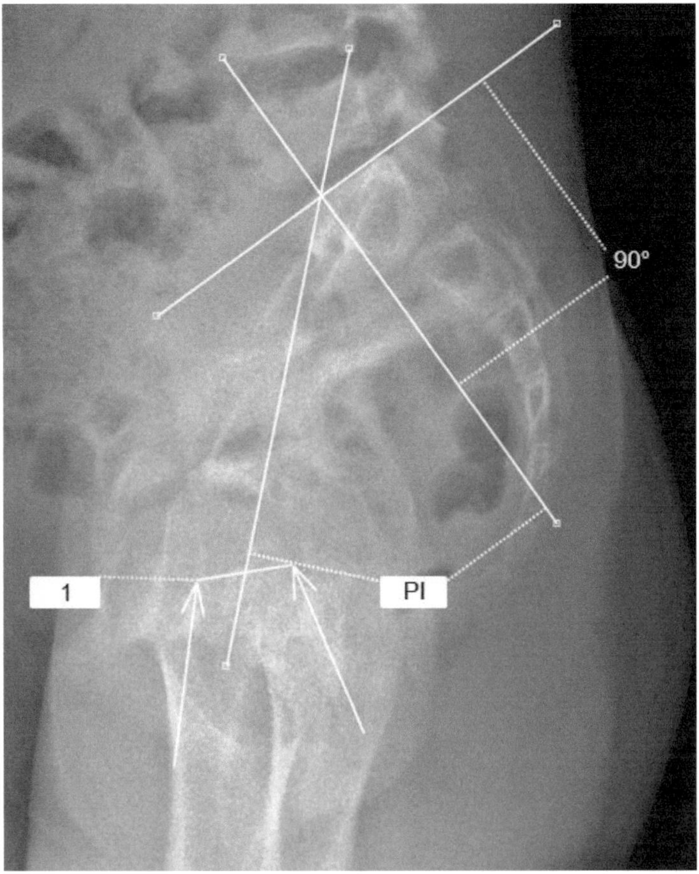

FIGURE 1 Pelvic incidence. *1* line between the centers of the femoral heads (arrows), *PI* pelvic incidence

Pelvic Tilt (PT)

The pelvic tilt (PT) is defined as the angle between two lines:

1. The vertical plane passing through the center of the femoral heads.
2. The line between the center of the superior endplate of S1 and the center of the femoral heads.

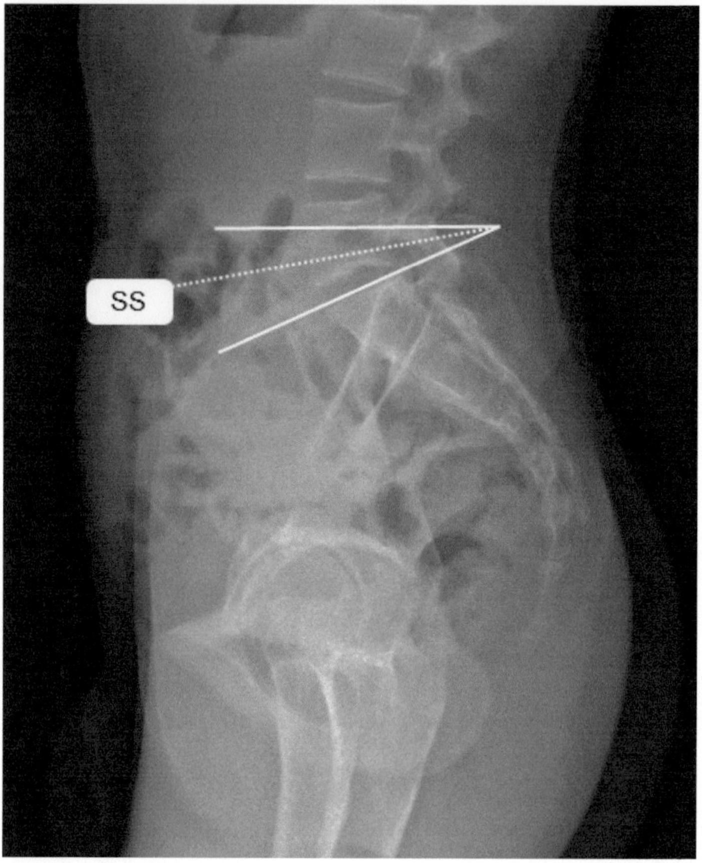

FIGURE 2 Sacral slope

If the femoral heads are not perfectly superimposed, the reference point is set midway between the lines connecting the center of the femoral heads.

The value of the PT may vary depending on the patient's position.

Normal values [8]:

- Between 3 and 8 years old: 5.5 ± 7.6 °.
- Between 8 and 18 years old: 7.7 ± 8.3 ° (Fig. 3).

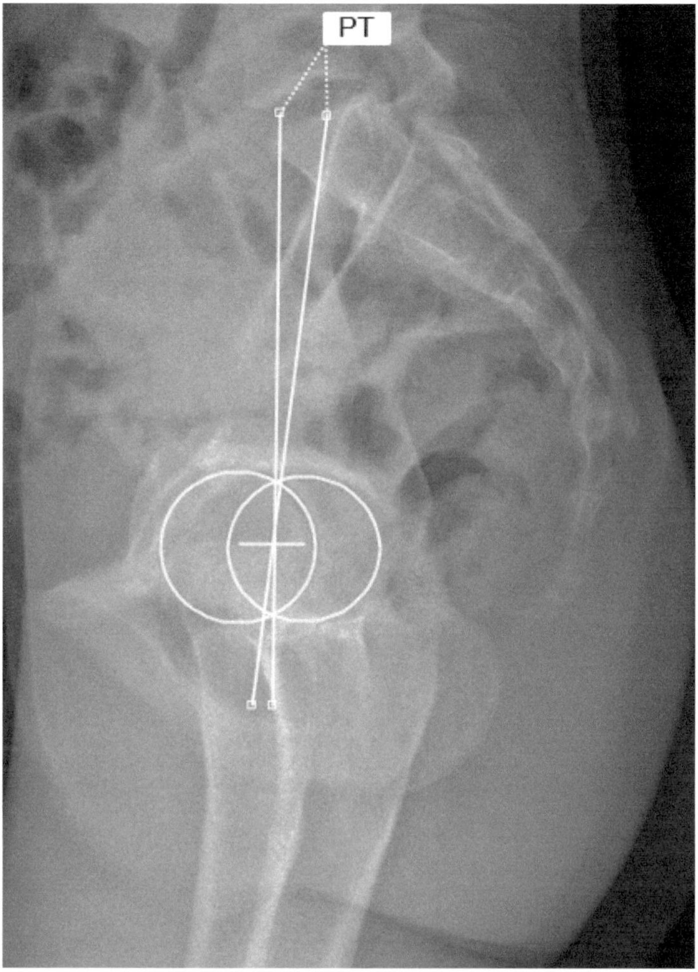

FIGURE 3 Pelvic tilt

Pelvic Obliquity (PO)

On the coronal images of the pelvis, the pelvic obliquity corresponds to the rotation of the pelvis in the coronal plane. It is the distance between two lines (measured on a line perpendicular to lines 1 and 2):

- Line 1 drawn horizontally across the most superior aspect of one acetabulum.
- Line 2 drawn horizontally across the most superior aspect of the other acetabulum.

Abnormal PO may have supra-pelvic causes such as scoliosis or infra-pelvic causes such as hip contracture, limb amputation (with prosthesis), and lower limb length discrepancy [9] (Fig. 4).

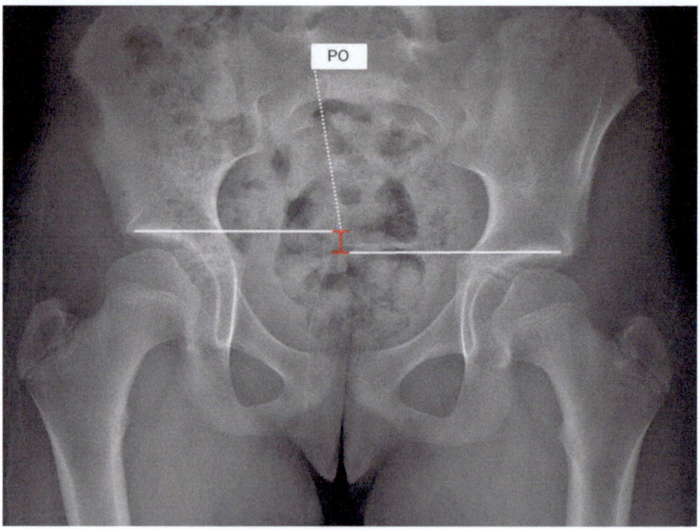

FIGURE 4 Pelvic obliquity

Pelvis axial rotation (2)	0°	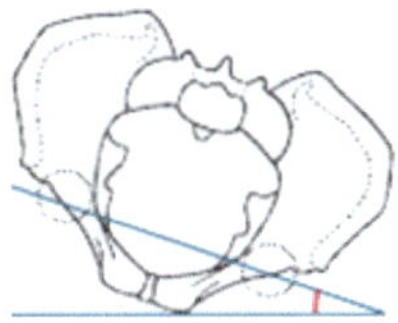

FIGURE 5 Example of the axial rotation of the pelvis as provided by the SterEOS report

Axial Rotation of the Pelvis (ARP)

The axial rotation of the pelvis is measured on 3D reconstruction and defined according to the coronal plane and measured between two lines:

1. The radiologic frontal plane (defined by the EOS acquisition planes).
2. The line between the centers of the two acetabula.

This measurement may be performed using the SterEOS® system [10] (Fig. 5).

Spine Measurements

Vertebral Numbering

When describing a spinal deformity, it is essential to use a consistent method for vertebral numbering. Cervical vertebrae are seldom involved in spinal deformities. By definition, a thoracic vertebra is associated with the presence of ribs [11]. However, radiologically, a very small rib cannot be distinguished from a small transverse process. Moreover, normal variants such as extra pairs of ribs exist. Therefore, it is sometimes impossible to number spinal vertebrae accurately, in which case an arbitrary choice is made and must be clearly mentioned in the report. Care must also be taken to always use the same numbering as in previous examinations [11].

Coronal Balance

Coronal balance is evaluated by measuring the distance between two lines, the CSVL (central sacral vertical line) and the C7 plumb line, as follows:

1. C7 plumb line: is drawn vertically from the central point of C7 downward.
2. CSVL: is drawn vertically from the central point of S1 upward.
   The coronal balance is mainly performed to assess spinal deviation in adolescent idiopathic scoliosis. Idiopathic scoliosis generally has a right curvature, and a left curve should be evaluated by MR to assess potential underlying issues.

C7-Central Sacral Line (CSL)

The C7-central sacral line (CSL) is the distance between two lines in the frontal plane:

1. A vertical line drawn from the central point of C7 (C7 plumb line).
2. A line drawn vertically from the central point of S1 upward (CSVL).

Balance is abnormal if the CSL is greater than 2 cm.

A negative value is measured when the vertical plumb line deviates to the left; a positive value is measured when the vertical plumb line deviates to the right (Fig. 6).

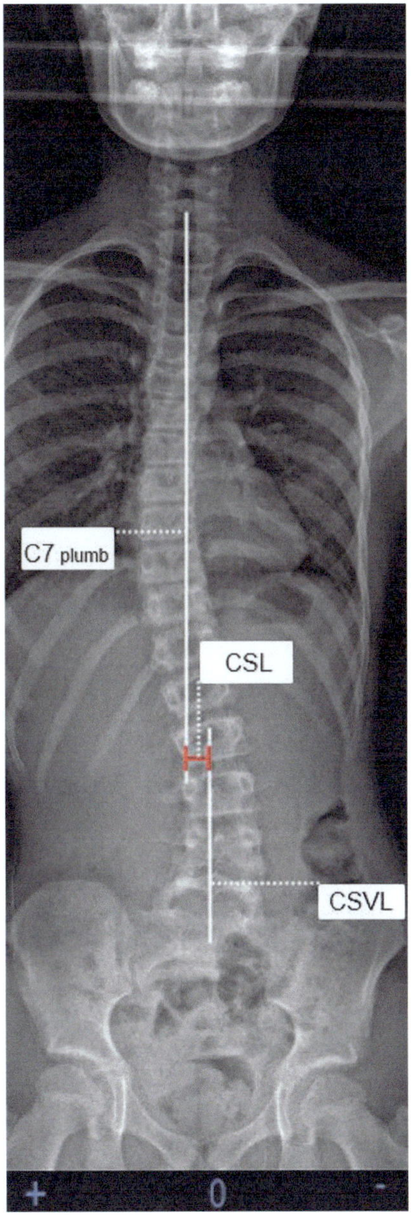

FIGURE 6 C7-central sacral line

Cobb Angle

The Cobb angle is defined as the angle between the two tangents drawn along the superior endplate of the superior end vertebra and the inferior endplate of the inferior end vertebra, in the scoliotic curve. The superior or inferior borders of the pedicles can be used instead of the endplates if these are not clearly visible.

The end vertebrae are those most tilted. The apex of the curve is the disk or the vertebra most horizontal and laterally placed from the center of the vertebral column (Figs. 7 and 8).

Scoliosis is defined as a lateral spinal curvature with a Cobb angle of ≥10°.

Diurnal variations of the Cobb angle up to 5° are possible [12].

A progressive curve that requires management is defined by a Cobb angle increase of 5° or more between consecutive radiographic examinations. The same measurements (same vertebrae) should be used for the follow-up examinations [12].

Structural curves, described by their location, lack normal flexibility and are termed as major (if they have the largest Cobb measurement) or minor. Minor curves can be structural or nonstructural [13]. Pelvic obliquity >2 cm must be corrected to measure the Cobb angles [13].

Lateral Flexion (Bending) Radiographs

If a curve cannot be corrected with ipsilateral bending to a curve <25° and/or kyphosis >20°, it is considered structural [13].

In-Brace Measurements

The measurements performed in brace should evaluate the curvature corrected by the brace with the same reference vertebrae as the image without brace.

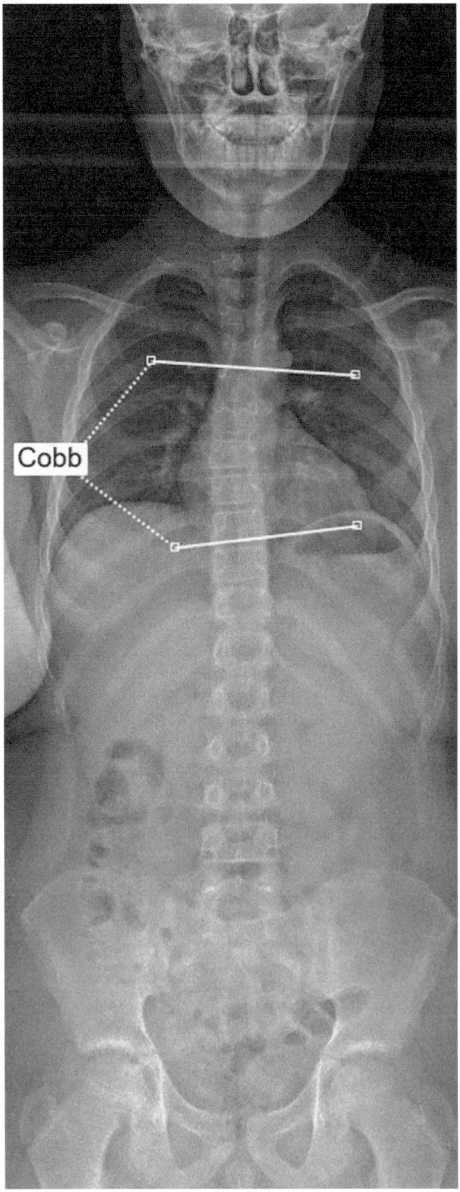

FIGURE 7 Cobb angle

Scoliosis parameters (1)		Value	
Curve (T7-T9-T12)	Cobb (T7-T9-T12)	**46°**	
	Axial rotation of apical vertebra T9	**-2°**	
Curve (T12-L1-L4)	Cobb (T12-L1-L4)	**40°**	
	Axial rotation of apical vertebra L1	**21°**	

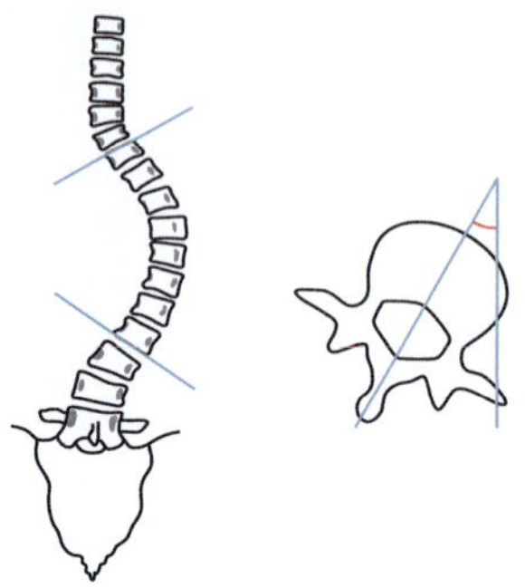

FIGURE 8 Example of spine measurements of the Cobb angles in a SterEOS report

If the curvature of the spine increases by more than 5° during brace treatment or if it is over 40° at skeletal maturity, the diagnosis of bracing failure is made [14].

In-brace correction <25% is a predictive factor of brace treatment failure in patients with double curves [14].

Sagittal Balance

Sagittal Vertical Axis (SVA) and CAM Plumb Line

On the sagittal view, C7 plumb line is a vertical line drawn downward from the central point of the C7 vertebral body. The C7 plumb line is the reference to measure the sagittal vertical axis (SVA). The SVA is evaluated by measuring the distance between the posterosuperior aspect of the S1 vertebral body and C7 plumb line. A positive SVA is defined by a C7 plumb line anterior to the posterosuperior margin of S1 and a negative sagittal balance by a C7 plumb line posterior to the posterosuperior margin of S1. A distance >2 cm is considered abnormal. C7 plumb line tends to move backward from childhood to adulthood. Progressive forward displacement of C7 plumb line in children should raise a suspicion for the risk of spinal pathology [8].

The Center of Acoustic Meati (CAM) is defined by the distance between the vertical line drawn from the center of acoustic meati (CAM plumb line) and the center of acetabula. The CAM is positive if the CAM plumb line is anterior to the acetabula. The CAM plumb line is useful for the clinical and radiological evaluation of the sagittal balance, even if it does not coincide with the gravity line. Normative CAM values in children have not been established yet [15] (Fig. 9).

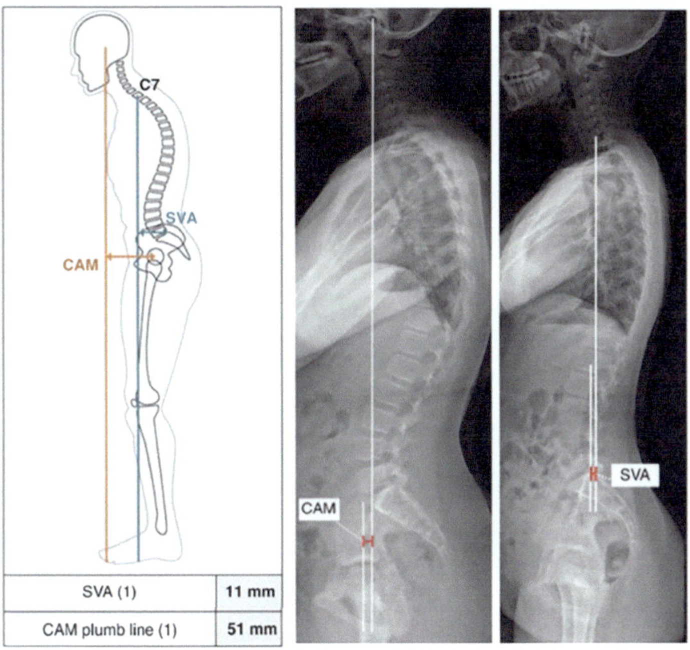

FIGURE 9 Example of SVA and CAM plumb line provided in a SterEOS report

Spino-Sacral Angle (SSA)

The spino-sacral angle (SSA) corresponds to an angle measured between two lines:

- A line drawn from the central point of C7 to the midpoint of the superior endplate of S1.
- A line tangent to the endplate of S1.

Normal SSA values are 130° ± 10° in subjects aged 3–10 years and 133° ± 8° in subjects between 10 and 18 years [8] (Fig. 10).

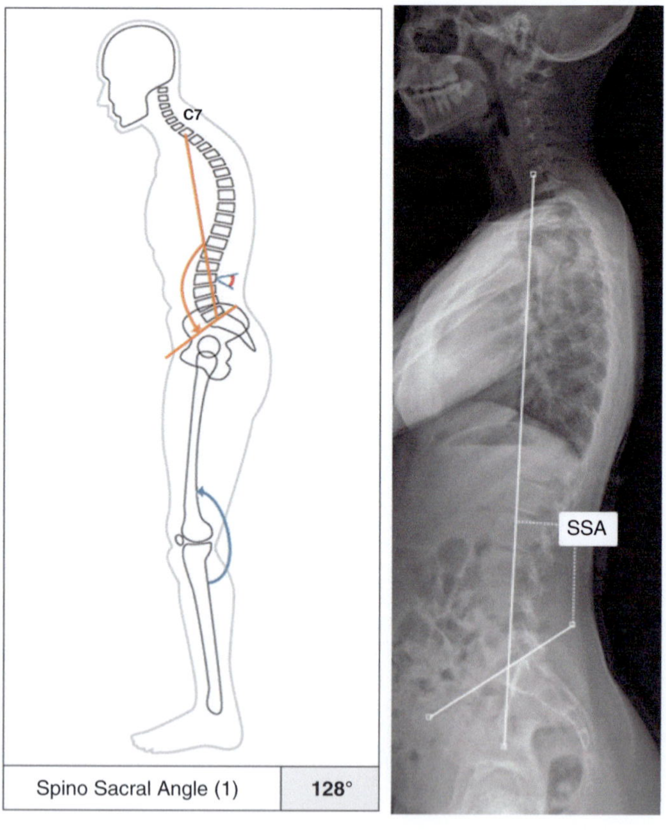

FIGURE 10 Example of SSA provided in a SterEOS report

T9 Tilt or T9 Sagittal Offset

In the sagittal plane, the T9 tilt (also know as Duval-Beaupère angle) is the angle formed by two lines (Fig. 11):

- A line between the central point of the two femoral heads and the central point of T9.
- A vertical line drawn upward from the central point of the two femoral heads.

This angle is positive when the hip axis lies in front of the T9 vertebral center. There are no published values for children. However, its normal value is 11.3 ± 3.52 in young adults and it is considered relatively stable during life [16, 17].

Thoracic Kyphosis (TK) and Lumbar Lordosis (LL)

The thoracic kyphosis (TK) and lumbar lordosis (LL) are measured by Cobb angles (Fig. 12). By convention, kyphosis is a positive (+) measurement and lordosis is a negative (−) measurement.

The TK is the angle measured between the superior endplate of T1 and the inferior endplate of T12. Its theoretical value is 0.75 x L1-S1 lordosis. T1–T4 represents only 8–10° of the overall kyphosis. For this reason, when it is impossible to visualize properly the first thoracic vertebra, it is acceptable to measure the TK between T5 and T12. Normal values are comprised between 10° and 40°.

The LL is the angle measured between the superior endplate of L1 and the inferior endplate of L5.

When operating a scoliosis, the most important thing for the surgeon is to preserve the sagittal balance. After spine fixation, one of the major complications is the junctional syndrome, occurring generally in the first months after surgery. It is defined as an increase in the proximal kyphosis of ≥10°, which is the angle measured between the inferior endplate of the first instrumented vertebra and the superior endplate of the second vertebra above it [18, 19].

3D Images

An added advantage offered by the EOS compared to conventional radiographs is to allow 3D analysis (Figs. 11, 12, and 13).

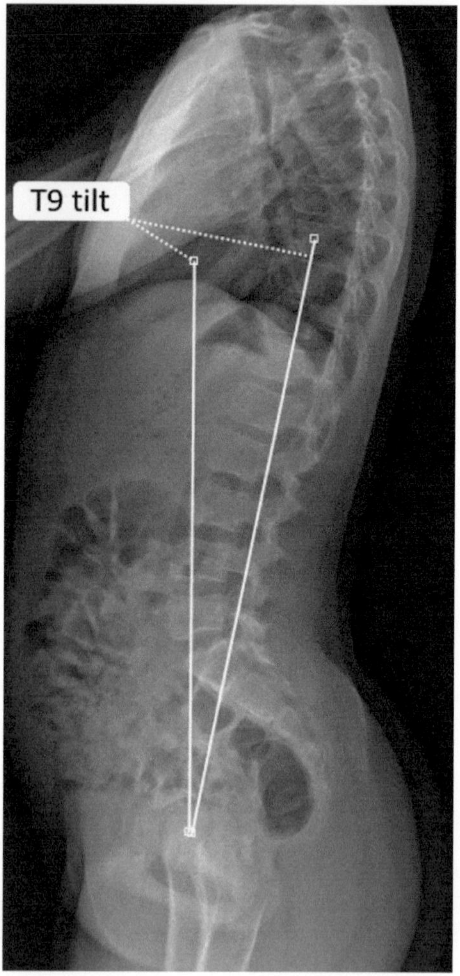

FIGURE 11 T9 tilt

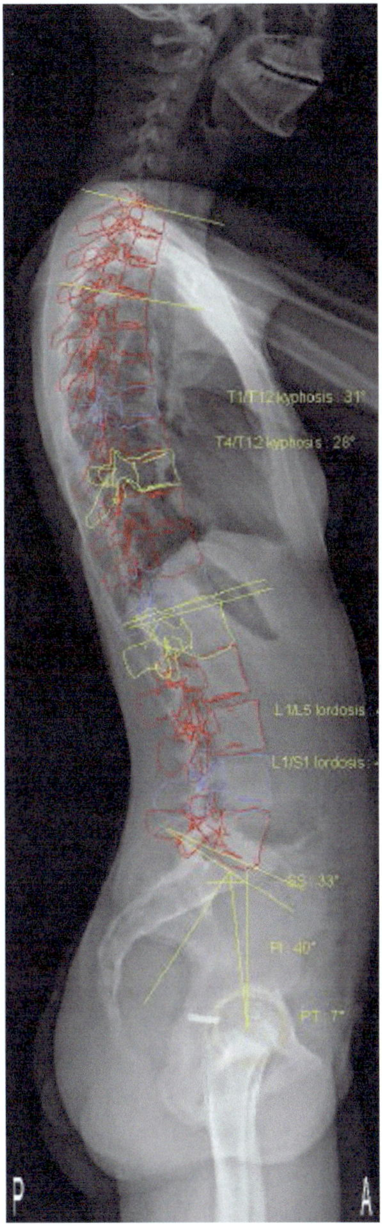

FIGURE 12 Thoracic kyphosis and lumbar lordosis

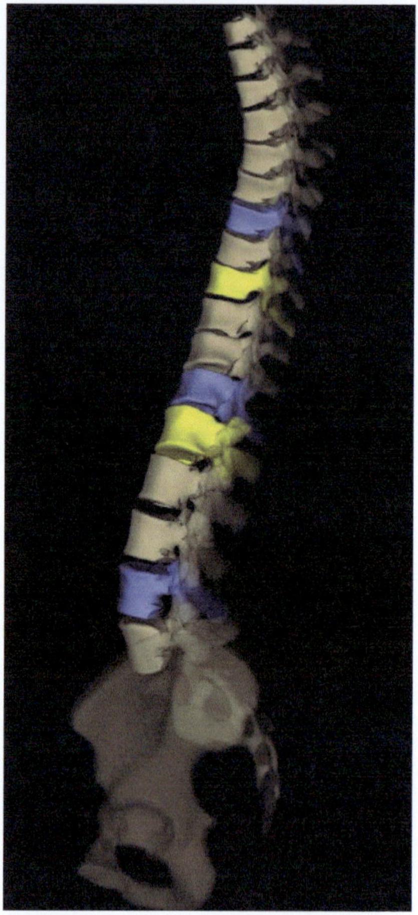

FIGURE 13 Example of a spine 3D reconstruction provided in a SterEOS report (lateral view)

Measurements of pelvic position were shown to be accurate and reliable with EOS. Reconstructed 3D images are within 1.1 mm ($\mp$ 0.2 mm) when compared to CT scan images. However, because these 3D reconstructions are based on standard bone models, they cannot be performed in cases of vertebral malformations, and they are not suitable for analyzing the ossification of the iliac apophysis (Risser classification) [20, 21] (Figs. 14 and 15).

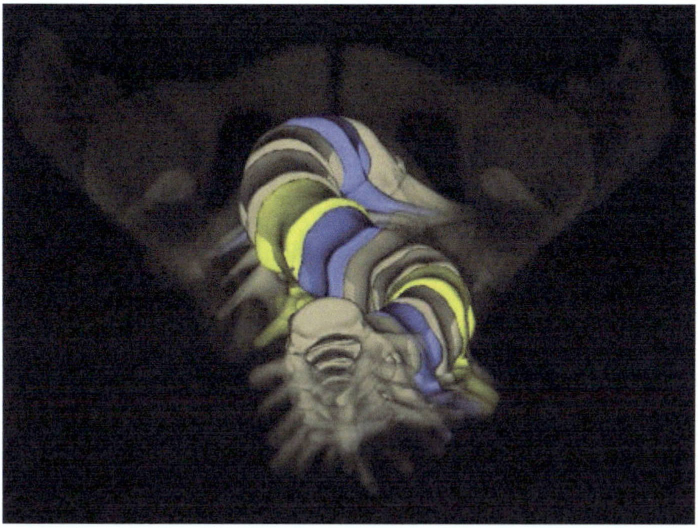

FIGURE 14 Example of a spine 3D reconstruction provided in a SterEOS report (cranio-caudal view)

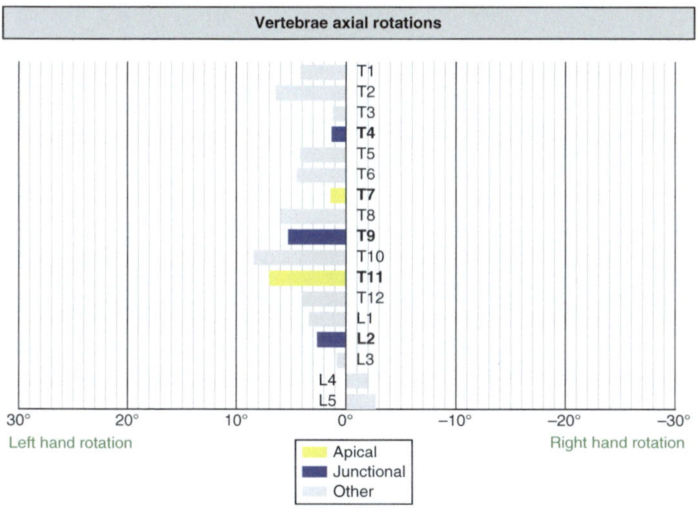

FIGURE 15 The diagram provides the axial rotation of the vertebrae calculated in relation to the pelvis

Lower Limb Measurements

Due to the relative novelty of the EOS imaging, few studies are currently available on the lower limb anatomical parameters in normal pediatric individuals. In this section, 16 lower limb measurements derived from EOS imaging are described.

1. Femoral Mechanical Axis Length [cm]: distance between the central point of the femoral head (A) and the midpoint of the distal femoral joint surface (B) (Figs. 16 and 17).
2. Tibial Mechanical Axis Length [cm]*: the distance between the midpoint of the intercondylar eminence (point C) and the midpoint of the distal tibial surface at the ankle (point D) (Fig. 17).

Age group (in years)	MALE	FEMALE
4 - 6	27.0 ± 2.0	25.5 ± 2.8
7 - 8	30.7 ± 2.9	30.6 ± 2.2
9 - 10	35.2 ± 2.2	35.9 ± 2.7
11 - 12	39.2 ± 3.0	39.6 ± 2.5
13 - 14	43.2 ± 2.2	40.9 ± 2.4
15 - 16	43.7 ± 2.5	41.2 ± 2.2

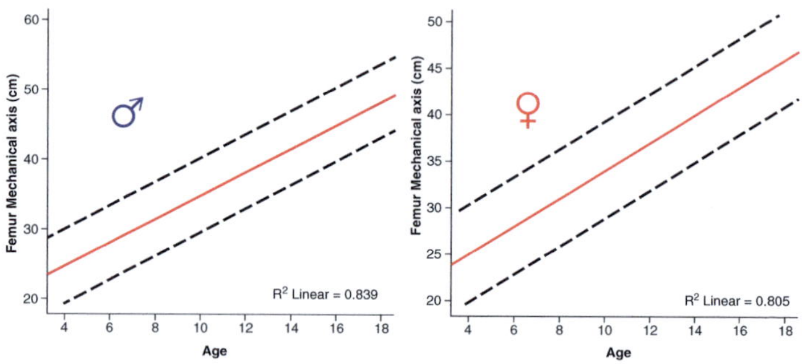

FIGURE 16 Adapted from Szuper et al. [22]

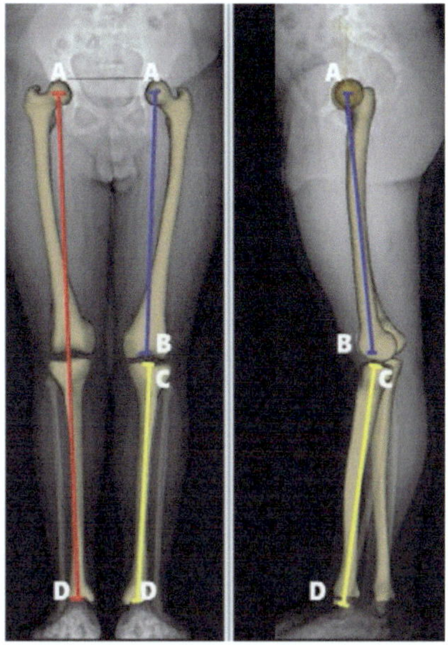

FIGURE 17 Lower limb axis

3. Functional Length of the Lower Limb [cm]*: the distance between points A and D (Fig. 17).
4. Anatomical Length of the Lower Limb [cm]*: the sum of the distance AB + CD (Fig. 17).

*At the time of writing, there are no published EOS imaging studies on the parameters described in points 2, 3 and 4.

5. Femoral Head Diameter [mm] (Fig. 18):
6. Femoral Offset [mm]: the distance between the central point of the femoral head and the line drawn through the femoral diaphysis axis are presented in the table below and in Fig. 19 (red line).

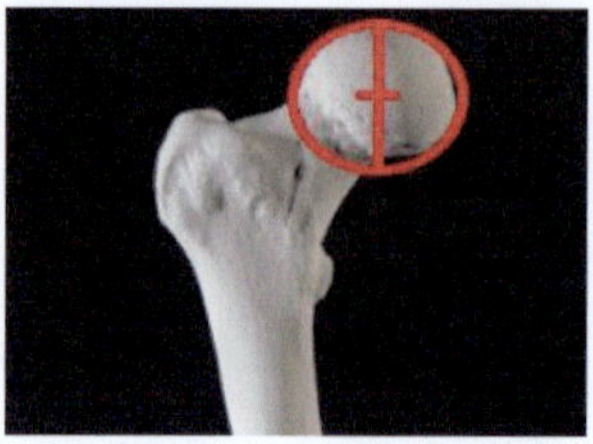

Age group (in years)	MALE	FEMALE
4 - 6	29.4 ± 2.5	27.7 ± 3.0
7 - 8	32.4 ± 2.8	32.1 ± 2.4
9 - 10	36.4 ± 2.6	36.7 ± 2.8
11 - 12	40.7 ± 3.6	39.9 ± 2.7
13 - 14	44.1 ± 2.9	40.7 ± 2.6
15 - 16	46.1 ± 2.7	41.3 ± 2.3

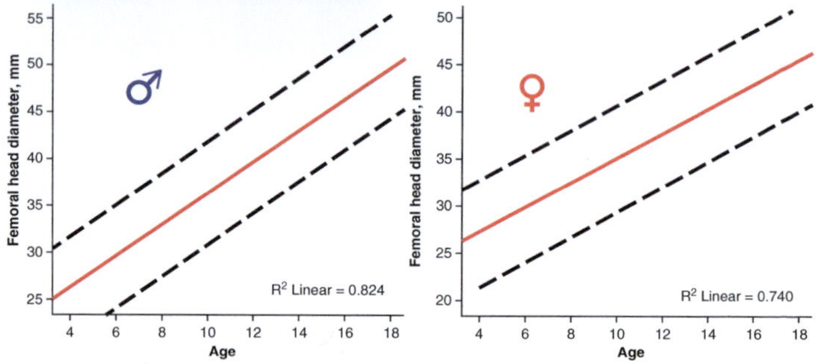

FIGURE 18 Adapted from Szuper et al. [22]

7. Femoral Neck Length [mm]: distance measured between the central point of the femoral head and the line bisecting the proximal femoral diaphysis (Fig. 20) (red line).

8. Neck/Shaft Angle (NSA) [Degrees]: the angle between the axis of the femoral diaphysis and the axis of the femoral neck originating from the center of the femoral head on the frontal plane (Fig. 21).

9. Femoral Mechanical Angle (FMA) [Degrees]: the angle between the femoral mechanical axis and the posterior bicondylar tangential line of the femur (Fig. 22).

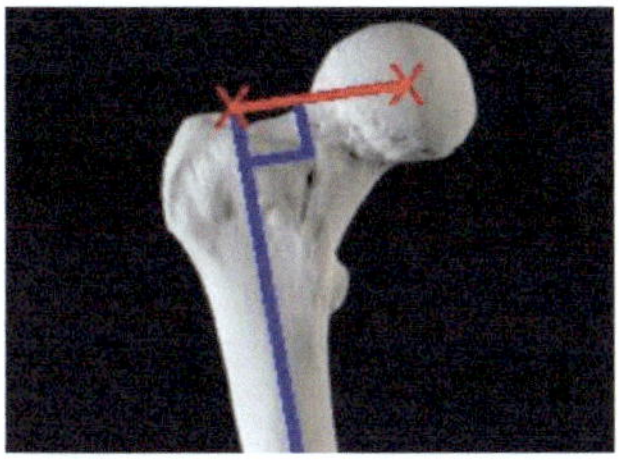

Age group (in years)	MALE	FEMALE
4 - 6	26.8 ± 3.8	25.5 ± 3.6
7 - 8	29.1 ± 3.4	29.0 ± 4.0
9 - 10	32.6 ± 4.2	32.5 ± 4.2
11 - 12	37.4 ± 4.5	36.8 ± 4.3
13 - 14	39.8 ± 4.7	37.5 ± 4.6
15 - 16	42.4 ± 4.9	37.9 ± 3.8

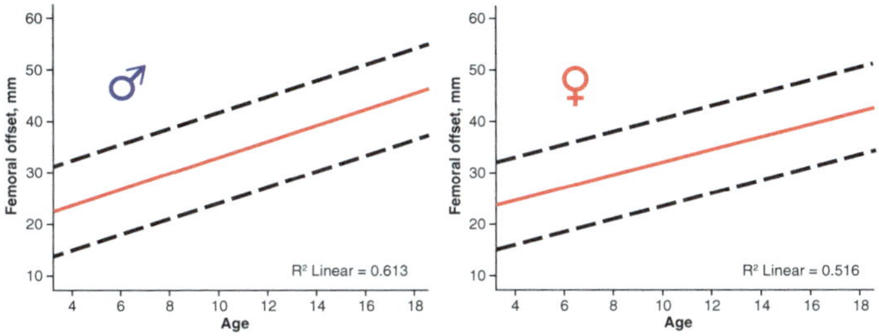

FIGURE 19 Adapted from Szuper et al. [22]

10. Tibial Mechanical Angle (TMA) [Degrees]: the angle between the tibial mechanical axis and the posterior bicondylar tangential line of the tibia (Fig. 23).

11. Mechanical Tibiofemoral Angle (FTA) [Degrees]: angle between the femoral and the tibial mechanical axis on the frontal plane. The varus and valgus deformation values of the knee are derived from this angle using the formula (180 °−FTA). Negative values mean varus, while positive values indicate valgus deformation (Fig. 24).

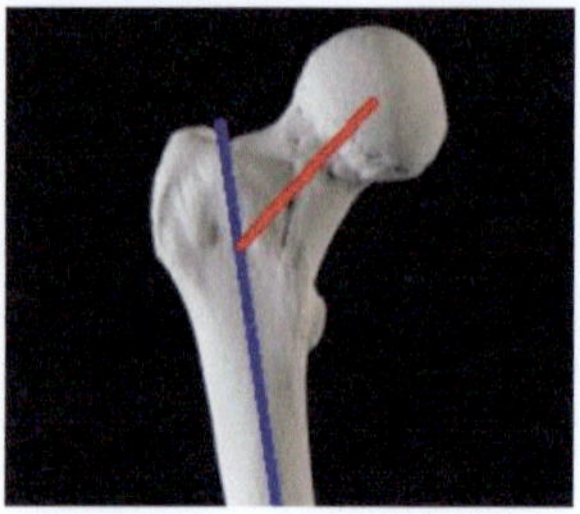

Age group (in years)	MALE	FEMALE
4 - 6	35.0 ± 4.0	32.8 ± 3.2
7 - 8	37.9 ± 3.4	37.2 ± 3.3
9 - 10	42.8 ± 3.3	42.9 ± 4.2
11 - 12	47.3 ± 4.3	46.8 ± 4.1
13 - 14	50.7 ± 4.1	48.2 ± 3.9
15 - 16	52.9 ± 4.3	48.1 ± 3.5

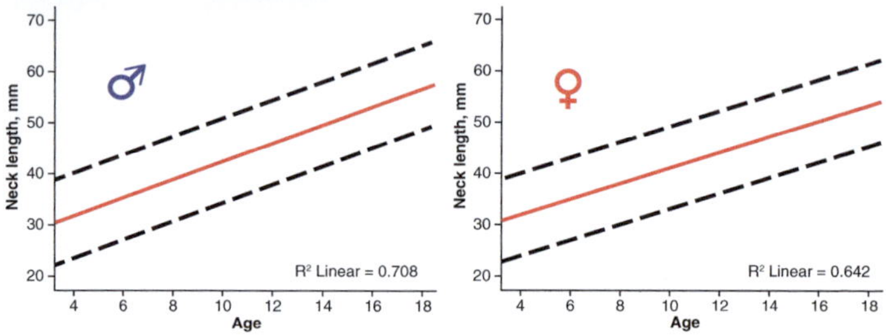

Figure 20 Adapted from Szuper et al. [22]

12. Hip-Knee-Shaft Angle (HKS) [Degrees]: angle between the mechanical femoral axis and the axis of the distal diaphysis on the frontal plane (Fig. 25).
13. Femoral Torsion Angle (FT) or Femoral Anteversion [Degrees]: angle defined between the femoral neck axis and the posterior bicondylar tangential line of the femur when projected on a plane orthogonal to the mechanical axis of the femur.

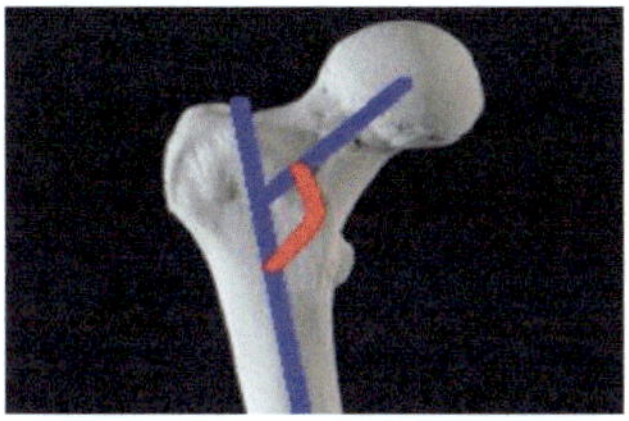

Age group (in years)	
4 - 6	130.4 ± 4.9
7 - 8	130.1 ± 5.3
9 - 10	130.9 ± 6.2
11 - 12	128.7 ± 4.5
13 - 14	129.2 ± 5.0
15 - 16	127.9 ± 4.3

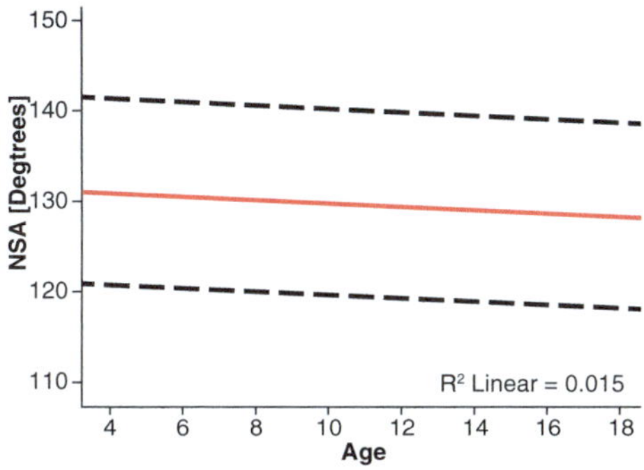

FIGURE 21 Adapted from Szuper et al. [22]

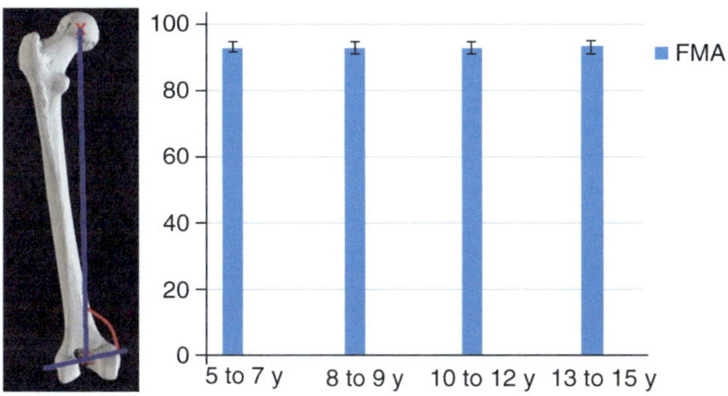

FIGURE 22 Adapted from Rampal et al. [23]

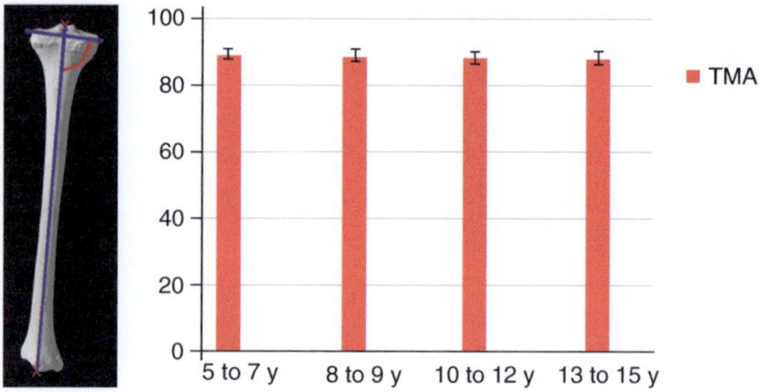

FIGURE 23 Adapted from Rampal et al. [23]

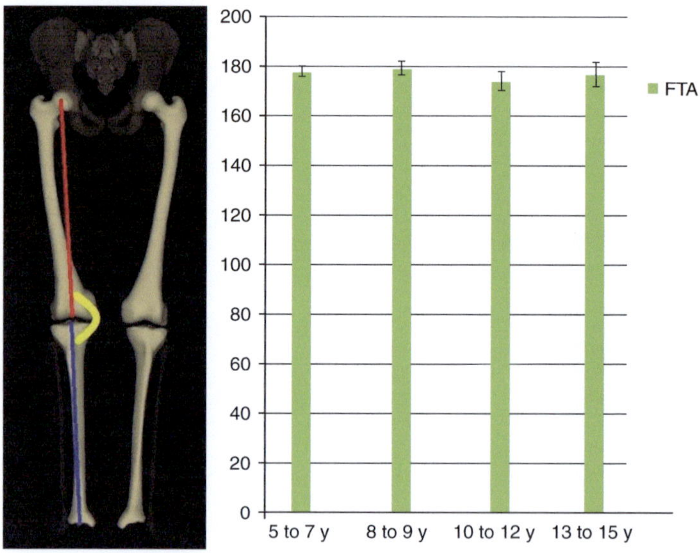

FIGURE 24 Adapted from Rampal et al. [23]

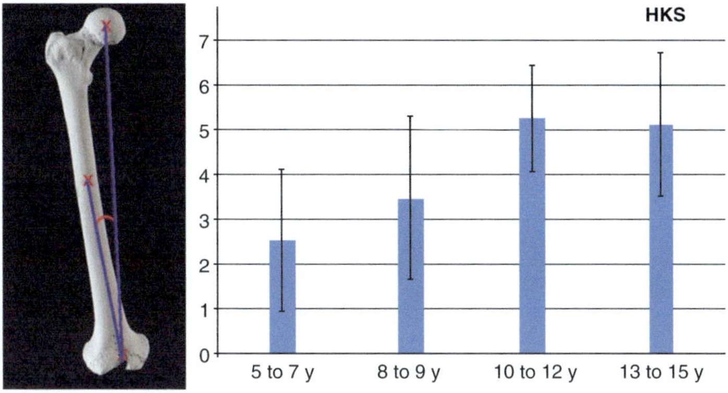

FIGURE 25 Adapted from Rampal et al. [23]

The FT is specific to the bipedal position of humans [24]. In humans, there is an early femoral torsion followed by a slow derotation that progresses throughout growth until adulthood (Fig. 26).

- The FT rapidly increases during the intrauterine life from the fourth to the ninth month. At birth, the FT is between 35° and 41° [25, 26].
- Later the distal femur tends to progressively rotate outward, and this angle decreases to the values described in Fig. 26.
- In adults, the normal value is 15.6 ± 6.7° [27].

14. Tibial Torsion Angle (TT) [Degrees]: angle defined between the posterior bicondylar tangential line of the tibia and the transmalleolar axis when projected on a plane orthogonal to the tibial mechanical axis.

This angle is usually positive in children, so the two malleoli are rotated relative to the tibia (Fig. 27).

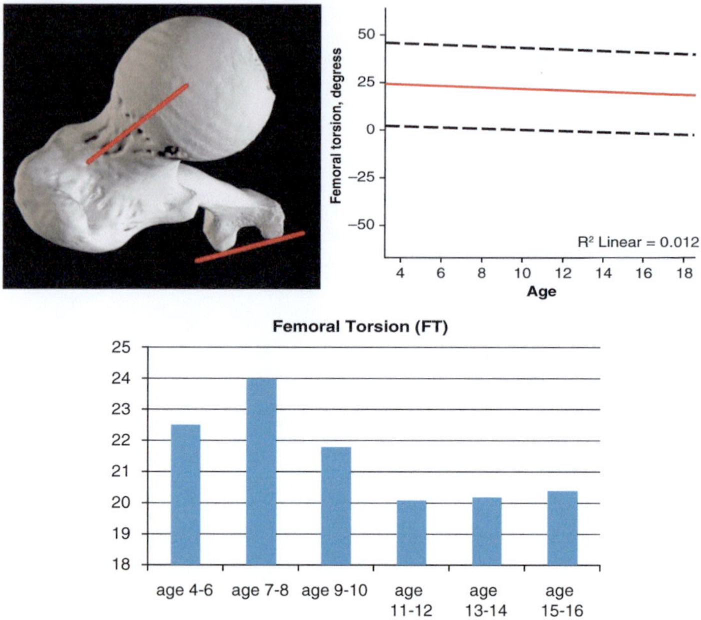

Figure 26 Adapted from Szuper et al. [22]

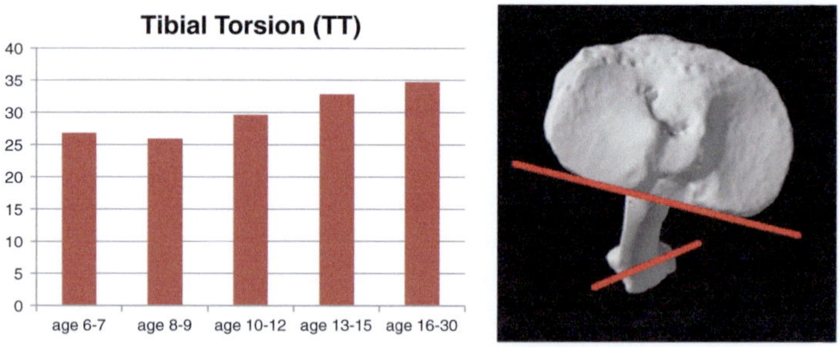

Figure 27 Adapted from Gaumétou et al. [28]

- The constraints of the fetus in utero are responsible for tibial deformation, causing a physiological internal TT, which will be from 2° to 10° during the first year of life and from 10° to 20° up to the age of 4 [25].
- Studies performed with EOS imaging have allowed us to reconstruct the evolution of TT in the pediatric age, as described in the values on Fig. 27.
- In adults, the average angle is 23 ± 5.1° [27].

15. Femorotibial Rotation (FTR) [Degrees]: the angle between the posterior bicondylar tangential line of the femur and the posterior bicondylar tangential line of the tibia when projected on an orthogonal plane to the femoral mechanical axis. If this angle is positive, then the tibia is externally rotated relative to the femur.

    To date, there are no published EOS imaging studies on this parameter of the lower limb in children (Fig. 28).
16. Sagittal Femorotibial Angle (SFTA) [Degrees]: angle between the mechanical axis of the femur and the mechanical axis of the tibia in the sagittal plane. The expected value in standing position is 180° (Fig. 29).

    The genu recurvatum is the hyperextension of the knee beyond 180°. The flexion of the knee occurs when the SFTA is less than 180°.

    The flexion/recurvatum is calculated with the formula 180° – STFA. Positive values of SFTA indicate flexion, and negative values indicate genu recurvatum.

    Values of recurvatum between 5° and 15° are considered physiological, and they are found in up to 40% of the population. A recurvatum beyond 15° is usually regarded as pathological [29].

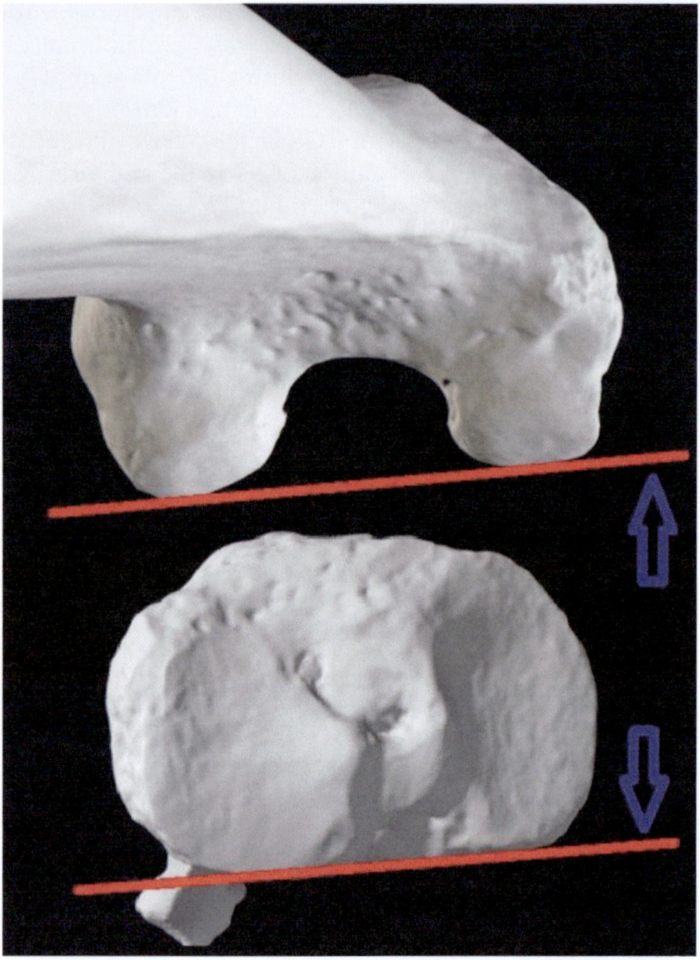

Figure 28 Measurement of femorotibial rotation (FTR)

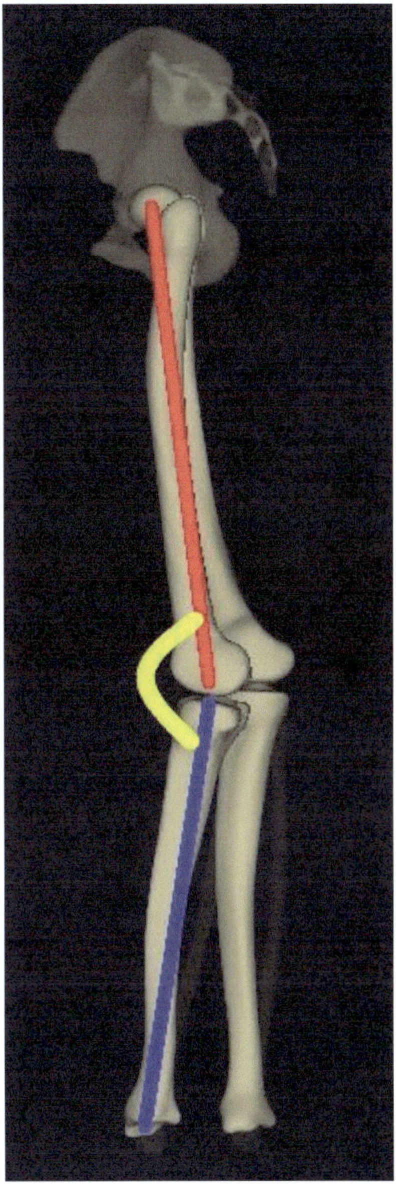

FIGURE 29 Measurement of the sagittal femorotibial angle (SFTA)

References

1. Wybier M, Bossard P. Musculoskeletal imaging in progress: the EOS imaging system. Joint Bone Spine. 2013;80(3):238–43. Epub 2012 Nov 22. https://doi.org/10.1016/j.jbspin.2012.09.018.
2. McKenna C, Wade R, Faria R, Yang H, Stirk L, Gummerson N, Sculpher M, Woolacott N. EOS 2D/3D X-ray imaging system: a systematic review and economic evaluation. Health Technol Assess. 2012;16(14):1–188. PMID: 22449757; PMCID: PMC4781036. https://doi.org/10.3310/hta16140.
3. Ilharreborde B, Dubousset J, Le Huec JC. Use of EOS imaging for the assessment of scoliosis deformities: application to postoperative 3D quantitative analysis of the trunk. Eur Spine J. 2014;23(Suppl 4):S397–405. Epub 2014 May 9. Erratum in: Eur Spine J. 2014 Jul;23 Suppl 4:S468. PMID: 24811688. https://doi.org/10.1007/s00586-014-3334-7.
4. Melhem E, Assi A, El Rachkidi R, Ghanem I, EOS(®). biplanar X-ray imaging: concept, developments, benefits, and limitations. J Child Orthop. 2016;10(1):1–14. Epub 2016 Feb 16. PMID: 26883033; PMCID: PMC4763151. https://doi.org/10.1007/s11832-016-0713-0.
5. Powell J, Gibly RF, Faulk LW, Carry P, Mayer SW, Selberg CM. Can EOS imaging substitute for conventional radiography in measurement of acetabular morphology in the young dysplastic hip? J Pediatr Orthop. 2020;40(6):294–9.
6. Legaye J, Duval-Beaupère G, Hecquet J, Marty C. Pelvic incidence: a fundamental pelvic parameter for three-dimensional regulation of spinal sagittal curves. Eur Spine J. 1998;7(2):99–103.
7. Bailey JF, Shefi S, Soudack M, Kramer PA, Been E. Development of pelvic incidence and lumbar lordosis in children and adolescents. Anat Rec. 2019;302(12):2132–9.
8. Mac-Thiong JM, Labelle H, Roussouly P. Pediatric sagittal alignment. Eur Spine J. 2011;20(Suppl 5):586–90.
9. Chan CYW. Pelvic obliquity in adolescent idiopathic scoliosis planned for posterior spinal fusion: a preoperative analysis of 311 lower limb axis films. J Orthop Surg. 2019;27(2):2309499019857250.
10. Rousseau MA, Brusson A, Lazennec JY. Assessment of the axial rotation of the pelvis with the EOS® imaging system: intra—and inter-observer reproducibility and accuracy study. Eur J Orthop Surg Traumatol. 2014;24(6):891–5.

11. O'Brien MF, Kuklo TR, Blanke KM, Lenke LG. Spinal deformity study group radiographic measurement manual. Memphis, TN: Medtronic Sofamar Danek; 2008. https://www.oref.org/docs/default-source/default-document-library/sdsg-radiographic-measuremnt-manual.pdf?sfvrsn=2.
12. Kim H, Kim HS, Moon ES, Yoon CS, Chung TS, Song HTS, et al. Scoliosis imaging: what radiologists should know. Radiographics. 2010;30(7):1823–42.
13. Lenke LG, Betz RR, Harms J, Bridwell KH, Clements DH, Lowe TG, et al. Adolescent idiopathic scoliosis: a new classification to determine extent of spinal arthrodesis. J Bone Joint Surg Am. 2001;83(8):1169–81.
14. van den Bogaart M, van Royen B, Haanstra TM, et al. Predictive factors for brace treatment outcome in adolescent idiopathic scoliosis: a best-evidence synthesis. Eur Spine J. 2019;28:511–25. https://doi.org/10.1007/s00586-018-05870-6.
15. Gangnet V, Pomero R, Dumas W, et al. Variability of the spine and pelvis location with respect to the gravity line: a three-dimensional stereoradiographic study using a force platform. Vital Surg Radiol Anat. 2003;25:424–33. https://doi.org/10.1007/s00276-003-0154-6.
16. Legaye J, Duval-Beaupere G. Sagittal plane alignment of the spine and gravity: a radiological and clinical evaluation. Acta Orthop Belg. 2005;71:213–20.
17. Sangondimath G, Mallepally AR, Marathe N, Salimath S, Chhabra HS. Radiographic analysis of the sagittal alignment of spine and pelvis in asymptomatic Indian population. Asian Spine J. 2022;16(1):107–18.
18. Le Huec JC, Thompson W, Moshinaly C, Barrey C, Faundez A. Sagittal balance of the spine. Eur Spine J. 2019;28:1889–905.
19. Mac-Thiong JM, Berthonnaud E, Dimar JR 2nd, Betz RR, Labelle H. Sagittal alignment of the spine and pelvis during growth. Spine (Phila Pa 1976). 2004;29(15):1642–7.
20. Kim JT, Lee DH, Lee HD, Shin HB, Park B, Park S, et al. Validity of the EOS-determined pelvic parameters and orientation with pelvic positional variation: a phantom study. Sci Rep. 2021;11(1):10468.
21. Glaser DA, Doan J, Newton PO. Comparison of 3-dimensional spinal reconstruction accuracy: biplanar radiographs with EOS versus computed tomography. Spine (Phila Pa 1976). 2012;37(16):1391–7.

22. Szuper K, et al. Three-dimensional quantitative analysis of the proximal femur and the pelvis in children and adolescents using an upright biplanar slot-scanning X-ray system. Pediatr Radiol. 2015;45(3):411–21. https://doi.org/10.1007/s00247-014-3146-2.
23. Rampal V, et al. Lower-limb lengths and angles in children older than six years: reliability and reference values by EOS® stereo-radiography. Orthop Traumatol Surg Res. 2018;104(3):389–95. https://doi.org/10.1016/j.otsr.2017.10.007.
24. Kinzinger H, Castiaux P. Les vices de torsion des membres inférieurs. Historique, évolution clinique. Acta Orthop Belg. 1977;43:379–470.
25. Chaudier P, Villa V, Neyre P. Traité EM Consulte podologie: anomalie de torsion du squelette. Podologie. 2015:13. https://doi.org/10.1016/S0292-062X(15)60422-6.
26. Gulan G, et al. Femoral neck anteversion: values, development, measurement, common problems. Coll Antropol. 2000;24(2):521–7.
27. Lobenhoffer P, Galla M, Agneskirchner JD. Rotational osteotomies of the femur and the tibia, from: osteotomies around the knee: indications, planning, surgical techniques using plate fixator. Stuttgart, New York.: Distributed by Thieme: Davos: AO Publishing; 2008.
28. Gaumétou E, et al. EOS analysis of lower extremity segmental torsion in children and young adults. Orthop Traumatol Surg Res. 2014;100(1):147–51. https://doi.org/10.1016/j.otsr.2013.09.010.
29. Demey G, Lustig S, Servien E, Neyret P. Genu recurvatum osseux. EMC-Appareil Locomoteur. 2013;5:0246–521.

MIX
Papier aus verantwortungsvollen Quellen
Paper from responsible sources
FSC® C105338

If you have any concerns about our products,
you can contact us on
ProductSafety@springernature.com

In case Publisher is established outside the EU,
the EU authorized representative is:
Springer Nature Customer Service Center GmbH
Europaplatz 3, 69115 Heidelberg, Germany

Printed by Libri Plureos GmbH
in Hamburg, Germany